Future M.D.

Future M.D.

Honest Advice from Medical Students for Medical School Applicants

Aashish R. Parikh

Writers Club Press

San Jose New York Lincoln Shanghai

Future M.D.
Honest Advice from Medical Students for Medical School Applicants

Writers Club Press
an imprint of iUniverse, Inc.

For information address:
iUniverse, Inc.
5220 S. 16th St., Suite 200
Lincoln, NE 68512
www.iuniverse.com

ISBN: 0-595-23058-X

Printed in the United States of America

To Ramesh and Chhaya Parikh, two of the most understanding and supportive parents, and Amy and Alay Parikh, my big sis and my baby brother. To Rachel, the love of my life.

Epigraph

Some patients, though conscious that their condition is perilous, recover their health simply through their contentment with the goodness of the physician.
—Hippocrates, 460-400 B.C.

CONTENTS

PREFACE

To cure sometimes, to relieve often, to comfort always.
—Anonymous, 15th Century or earlier

Future M.D. is written by medical students for future medical students. Bookstores are filled with medical school admissions books, but have you looked at the authors? Most of them have never applied to medical school themselves. If they did, it was twenty years ago. Much has changed since then and the competition gets stronger every year. When I applied to medical school, I read all of those books. Not a single one was written by a medical student. After having been through the admissions process, I realize that most books on the subject are not accurate at all. In fact, much of the advice is outdated and contains too many generalities. I have found the best advice for applying to medical school comes directly from people who have recently gone through the admissions process. There is no substitute for firsthand experience.

What makes our advice different from any other? We show exactly what it takes to get into medical school. This book is aimed at those who are serious about their career in medicine and are willing to do whatever it takes to gain admission. Included are tips to boost your GPA and make your application stand out above the thousands of others. This book lists the most frequently asked questions during the interview process and helps you develop good answers. It even mentions exactly what to wear to your interview and what questions you should ask. Real personal statements from current medical students are included, not necessarily suggestions of a premed advisor.

Almost all medical school admissions books include a section about rejection and what to do if this occurs to you. I always found these parts extremely disappointing and in my opinion serve no purpose for the serious applicant. Rather, it's important to keep a positive perspective in pursuing your goal of admission. If you fail to get in on your first try, apply again. I know plenty of doctors who had to do a year of research or got a Master's or a Ph.D. before going to medical school. I also know many physicians who went to foreign medical schools. Your goal is to become a physician, and that is exactly why this book is written.

Essentially, I have composed exactly the type of book I would love to have read before applying to medical school. *Future M.D.* is a compilation of my experiences through the process and the best advice I received from successful medical school applicants. I sincerely hope the reader will find its contents helpful and straightforward.

I wish you the best of luck in your exciting career in medicine!

Aashish R. Parikh

April 2002

LIST OF CONTRIBUTORS

Cristina Baseggio
Yale University School of Medicine
Class of 2005

Meghan R. Forster
University of Cincinnati College of Medicine
Class of 2004

Ajay V. Maker, M.D.
Yale University School of Medicine
Class of 2001

Alay R. Parikh
The University of Texas at Austin
Class of 2005

Chirayu J. Shah
Baylor College of Medicine
Class of 2005

INTRODUCTION

Medicine is neither a job nor a career; it is a life. Once you become a doctor, you have joined one of the noble professions. When you wake up in the morning, you will be a physician. When you go to sleep at night, you will be a physician. You will be a physician until the day you leave this earth. With this profession comes a great deal of expectation and responsibility. Not only is a physician liable for his own life, but also the lives of each and every patient he treats and counsels. You will find that patients tell you intimate details of their lives they wouldn't dare tell their spouses, parents, children, or clergy. The medical profession indeed requires a special type of human being.

A good physician treats not only the disease, but also serves as an aggressive advocate for his patients. A great physician has the ability to reach inside a patient's mind and body to see life from that perspective. Becoming a great physician takes a lifetime. No one expects you to have these attributes by day one of medical school, and that is exactly why you attend medical school for four years followed by an internship and residency.

When applying to medical school you will be asked countless times, "Why would anyone want to enter medicine, and these days?" We have all heard the phrase, "I want to help people." Even though this is a good reason, you can "help people" working at a grocery store or mowing lawns for a living. What separates medicine from other professions is the opportunity to have a true impact on the lives of others in a rewarding way, and it offers a tremendous opportunity for personal growth.

Unfortunately, some doctors enter the profession for reasons other than "to help." Money, respect and social status are different incentives, which can ultimately result in misery and are simply not worth it. Before applying to medical school, be sure you have the motivation and dedication to become a fine physician, one who will respect patients and be willing to learn for the rest of your life. You will learn from inside as well as outside the classroom and, more importantly, from your mistakes and the mistakes of others.

There is no simple formula for getting into medical school and there is no such thing as an ideal applicant. But what you can do is demonstrate exactly why you wish to become a physician in a lucid and succinct manner. You also must have the academic skills necessary to make it through medical school. Each year approximately 40,000 students apply for 16,000 medical school positions, and our goal here is to separate you from the other 24,000 applicants.

Finally, never let anyone tell you that you cannot do something; they're dead wrong. They're wrong because they don't know you and they don't know your motivations for becoming a physician. Never lose sight of your dreams and never forget that the mission of medicine is the relief of human suffering.

A Doctor's Education

The most essential part of a student's instruction is obtained…not in the lecture-room, but at the bedside. Nothing seen there is lost; the rhythms of disease are learned by frequent repetition; its unforeseen occurrences stamp themselves indelibly in the memory.
—Oliver Wendell Holmes, M.D.

Path to Becoming a Physician

Medical doctors receive one of the most arduous and lengthy education, training and licensing procedures before starting a practice. The path to becoming a physician usually starts with four years of undergraduate education followed by four years of medical school. Historically, medical school curricula are divided into two phases. The first two years of medical school are labeled "basic science or pre-clinical," in which the focus is placed on lectures and laboratory work. Courses taught during this time include anatomy, biochemistry, microbiology, pathology, pharmacology, and physiology. The third and fourth years of medical school involve working with patients under the guidance of senior doctors at a variety of teaching hospitals and clinics.

After graduating from medical school, doctors must complete 1 to 3 years of residency training, which makes them eligible to take their examination for a medical license. The strong majority of doctors continue onward to complete specialty training in a residency program. The length of training varies from specialty to specialty, ranging from 3 to 8 years. Following internships and residencies, doctors must pass additional examinations to become certified by a specialty board. The final frontier of medical education involves fellowships to develop expertise in a subspecialty. Fellowships typically last 1 to 2 years.

Doctors stay in touch with new medical developments and techniques by taking continuing medical education (CME) courses. Some states, professional organizations, and hospital medical staff require a certain number of CME credits to ensure the doctor's knowledge remains current.

Figure 1.1

Education & Training For A Physician

☑ **BACHELOR'S DEGREE** – four years of education at a college or university

☑ **MEDICAL DEGREE** – four years of education and training at an accredited medical school or school of osteopathic medicine

☑ **MEDICAL LICENSE** – all practicing doctors must have a license to practice medicine in the state(s) where they are working

☑ **SPECIALTY TRAINING** – doctors enter into a residency program for three to 8 years (specialty dependent) of professional training under the supervision of senior physicians

☑ **BOARD CERTIFICATION** – certification ensures that a doctor has been tested to assess his or her knowledge and experience in a specialty and is deemed qualified to provide patient care in that specialty

☑ **FELLOWSHIP** – some doctors pursue two or more years of additional training and in some specialty to become even more specialized in a particular field

☑ **CONTINUING MEDICAL EDUCATION (CME)** – doctors may continue to receive credit for continuing education

Source: The Journal of the American Medical Association. September 6, 2000

Medical School Curriculum

Currently, most medical schools offer a well-constructed curriculum providing a solid education in the basic sciences and clinical training. At the beginning of the 20th century, medical education in the United States varied greatly between different schools. The quality of medical schools was in question at the time and this concern prompted proposals to standardize premedical requirements, curriculum structure, educational formats, faculty qualifications, and methods of clinical training. In 1910 Abraham Flexner changed the landscape of medical education by outlining a unified model of medical education.

The first year of medical school focuses on learning everything that is "right" with the human body. Most students take anatomy, biochemistry, histology (microscopic anatomy), microbiology (immunology, virology, bacteriology, parasitology), physiology, and neuroscience (neuroanatomy). In addition, first-year students often learn how to interact with patients through an introduction course in clinical medicine. The second year is devoted to learning how and why things go "wrong" with the body and how one corrects these illnesses. During the second year students take pathology, pharmacology, genetics, behavioral science, and advanced clinical medicine. Some schools teach these courses separately or offer a system-based curriculum in which the year is divided by organ systems, such as cardiovascular, renal, reproductive, or other system.

The third and fourth years of medical school are devoted to required clinical clerkships and elective courses. The third year is typically divided by spending time in the following disciplines: family practice, internal medicine, neurology, obstetrics and gynecology, pediatrics, psychiatry, surgery, and the surgical subspecialties. The final year of medical school is the most flexible, in which students can take electives, rotate through programs they are interested in, participate in overseas medicine, and take time off to interview for residencies.

Figure 1.2

National Board Examinations

The National Board of Medical Examiners and the Federation of State Medical Boards require the United States Medical Licensing Examination (USMLE) to become eligible for a license to practice medicine. The USMLE consists of three separate exams spread out during your medical education. Steps 1 and 2 are taken before graduating from medical school. After receiving an MD or DO doctors must take Step 3, the final exam needed for licensure.

STEP 1	Typically taken between the second and third years of medical school.
	The Goal of the USMLE Step 1 is to test your understanding and application of important concepts in basic biomedical sciences.
STEP 2	Taken during the fourth year of medical school.
	The goal of Step 2 is to examine your ability to apply medical knowledge and clinical science needed for patient care.
STEP 3	Taken after graduating from medical school.
	The goal of Step 3 is to assess whether you can apply medical knowledge and clinical science required for general practice of medicine.

Source: National Board of Medical Examiners, 2002.

Allopathic and Osteopathic Medicine

Along with physicians receiving a doctor of medicine degree (M.D.), there are physicians who receive a doctor of osteopathy degree (D.O.). Both the M.D. and D.O. are required to pass the same state and national medical board examinations, and many complete their training in the same specialty programs.

Figure 1.3

The Eight Philosophical Osteopathic Precepts

■ The body is a unit. *

■ Structure and function are reciprocally interrelated. *

■ The body possesses self-regulatory mechanisms. *

■ The body has the inherent capacity to defend itself and repair itself. *

■ When normal adaptability is disrupted, or when environmental changes overcome the body's capacity for self-maintenance, disease may occur.

■ Movement of the body fluids is essential to the maintenance of health.

■ The nerves play a crucial part in controlling the fluids of the body.

■ There are somatic components to disease that are not only manifestations of disease but also are factors that contribute to maintenance of the diseased state.

* Original precepts developed in 1953 at the Kirksville College of Osteopathic Medicine

Source: *The Journal of the Osteopathic Association, September 1981*

Figure 1.4

Requirements/Training for Allopathic (M.D.) & Osteopathic (D.O.) Physicians

	Allopathic (M.D.)	Osteopathic (D.O.)
PREMEDICAL REQUIREMENTS	Biology (8 hours) Physics (8 hours) Inorganic Chemistry (8 hours) Organic Chemistry (8 hours) English (6 hours) Calculus (one semester) MCAT Score	Biology (8 hours) Physics (8 hours) Inorganic Chemistry (8 hours) Organic Chemistry (8 hours) English (6 hours) Calculus (one semester) MCAT Score
MEDICAL SCHOOL	Four Years	Four Years
INTERNSHIP	Three tracks are available: Medicine, Surgery or a Transitional Year	The AOA suggests an osteopathic Rotating Year in a AOA approved site (either MD or DO site)
RESIDENCY	Three to seven years followed by an optional fellowship	Three to seven years followed by an optional fellowship
LICENSING	Requirements Vary by State Call the AMA for more information	Requirements Vary by State Call the AOA for more information

Source: The Student Doctor Network, 2002

For more information, contact:

American Medical Association (AMA)
515 N. State Street
Chicago, IL 60610
(312) 464-5000
www.ama-assn.org

American Osteopathic Association (AOA)
142 E. Ontario Street
Chicago, IL 60611
(800) 621-1777
www.aoa-net.org

While there may be perceived differences between the M.D. and the D.O., the allopathic (M.D.) and osteopathic (D.O.) healers are both physicians. They both treat and counsel patients about health issues, and hopefully provide a healing touch. Some problems lie with past biases of the M.D. against the D.O. I'm really not sure why, but it's like being on a baseball team with all right-handers and suddenly a left-handed person starts to play, and plays well at that. Another analogy is comparing two different brands of cola. They both do the same thing, provide refreshment, but one may have a slightly different mix of ingredients. My own pediatrician was a D.O. and I couldn't have cared less about his type of degree. The only thing I cared about was that he was nice and helped me feel better when I was sick. If you really want to help patients, attending an allopathic or osteopathic medical school is a secondary concern, not the primary motivator.

For one reason or another, many students shy away from applying to both types of schools. But I think in doing so, you limit your chances of getting an acceptance letter. When the time came for me to apply to medical school, I sent applications to both M.D. and D.O. schools. I had a friend in college who didn't, and he actually made fun of me for applying to osteopathic schools. It's funny how life plays out and seems somewhat Shakespearean. I received an acceptance letter (from an allopathic school) before anyone else, and he received no letters. He ended up having to work for a year and then found the wisdom to apply to both types of schools. Eventually he went to an osteopathic medical college. Basically I'm saying do not allow any sort of arrogance to get in the way of becoming a physician. Medicine has no more room for it!

Graduate Medical Education: Internships and Residencies

The Intern: Within the medical chain of command, the intern is the person having just graduated from medical school working in residence at a teaching hospital. Internships (Post Graduate Year 1, or PGY-1) provide a transition phase between the medical student and the resident. This is when interns can sharpen their diagnostic skills and become an integral part of a medical team comprised of residents and attending physicians. Interns are allowed to write prescriptions at teaching facilities but not outside (they can't yet phone in a prescription to the local drug store). At the conclusion of this first year of residency, an intern sits for Step 3 of the USMLE, and now he or she is eligible to receive a license to practice medicine.

The Resident: After completing the grueling year of internship, the intern moves up the ladder and becomes a resident, part of the house staff (PGY-2, and higher). The resident's responsibility is to work directly with attending physicians to develop and carry treatment orders for patients. Many residents also find time to teach interns and medical students. Although many people may believe residents no longer have to put in long hours at the hospital, they do. I have seen situations where residents have not slept for days, but you should see residency as just another obstacle to cross before becoming a board certified physician.

Description of Medical Specialties

ANESTHESIOLOGY
To monitor and deliver analgesic medication to patients during operative procedures as well as management of patients suffering from chronic pain conditions.
Length of Residency: 4 years
Fellowships (1 to 2 additional years of training):
Cardiac Anesthesiology, Critical Care, Pain Management, Pediatric Anesthesiology, OB/GYN Anesthesiology, Vascular Anesthesiology, Neurosurgical Anesthesiology, Ambulatory Anesthesiology
Median Income: $225,000 per annum

DERMATOLOGY

Diagnose and treat disorders of the skin and mucous membranes.

Length of Residency: 4 years

Fellowships (1 additional year of training):

Dermatological Immunology/Diagnostic and Laboratory, Dermatopathology, Immunology, Dermatology Research

Median Income: $190,000 per annum

DIAGNOSTIC RADIOLOGY

Reading and diagnostic interpretation of various imaging modalities, such as radiographs, CT, MRI, ultrasound, and mammograms. In addition, radiologists also perform interventional procedures such as embolization and angioplasty.

Length of Residency: 5 years

Fellowships (1 to 2 additional years of training):

Neuroradiology, Vascular / Interventional Radiology, Mammography, Musculoskeletal Radiology, Pediatric Radiology, Body Imaging, Chest Radiology, CT, MRI, Ultrasonography, Nuclear Medicine

Median Income: $260,000 per annum

EMERGENCY MEDICINE

This medical specialty focuses on the rapid evaluation, work-up, and care of patients who are acutely ill or injured.

Length of Residency: 3 to 4 years

Fellowships (1 to 3 additional years of training):

Hospital / ER Administration (1 year), Disaster Medicine (2 years), EMS (1-2 years), Medical Education (1 year), Pediatric Emergency Medicine (2-3 years), Toxicology (1-2 years), Sports Medicine (1 year)

Median Income: $175,000 per annum

FAMILY PRACTICE

Provide primary medical care for the diagnosis, treatment, and prevention of conditions affecting patients of all ages.

Length of Residency: 3 years

Fellowships (1 to 2 additional years of training):

Adolescent Medicine (2 years), Faculty Development (1 year), Geriatric Medicine (1-2 years), Preventative Medicine (1-2 years), Research (1 year), Rural Medicine (1 year), Sports Medicine (1 year), Substance Abuse (1 year)

Median Income: $125,000 per annum

GENERAL SURGERY

Diagnosis and treatment (conservative versus operative) of a variety of abdominal as well as soft tissue conditions.

Length of Residency: 5 years

Fellowships (1 to 3 additional years of training):

General Surgery Research (2 years), Cardiothoracic Surgery (2-3 years), Colorectal Surgery (1-2 years), Pediatric Surgery (2 years), Surgical Critical Care (2 years), Surgical Oncology (1-2 years), Transplant Surgery (2-3 years), Vascular Surgery (1-2 years), Hand Surgery (1 year), Plastic Surgery (2-3 years)

Median Income: $200,000 per annum

INTERNAL MEDICINE

Providing medical care for adult and geriatric patients in the hospital and in the office. Diagnosis and treatment of acute and chronic medical illnesses. Also emphasizes preventative measures such as regular medical checkups and screening tests, as well as healthy lifestyle habits. Often described as an "adult's pediatrician."

Length of Residency: 3 years

Fellowships (1 to 3 additional years of training):

Sports Medicine (1 year), Cardiac Electrophysiology (1 year), Infectious Disease (2 years), Geriatric Medicine (2-3 years), Allergy and Immunology (2-3 years), Cardiology (3 years), Endocrinology (2 years), Gastroenterology (3 years), Hematology and Oncology (2-3 years), Nephrology (2 years), Pulmonary Medicine (2 years), Rheumatology (2 years), Critical Care Medicine (1-2 years), Internal Medicine Research (1-2 years)
Median Income: $140,000 per annum

NEUROLOGY
Diagnosis and treatment of nervous system disorders involving the brain, spinal cord, and other neuromuscular conditions, as well as the blood vessels that relate to them.
Length of Residency: 4 years
Fellowships (1 to 3 additional years of training):
Neurology Research (1-2 years), Critical Care Medicine (1-2 years), Clinical Neurophysiology (1 year), Pediatric Neurology (3 years)
Median Income: $160,000 per annum

NEUROSURGERY
Diagnosis as well as operative and nonoperative management of disorders affecting the brain, spinal cord, peripheral nervous system, vertebrae, and cerebral vasculature. Neurosurgeons also participate in critical care and rehabilitation of paraplegia as well as other neurologic disorders, including the management of chronic pain conditions.
Length of Residency: 6 to 7 years
Fellowships (1 to 3 additional years of training):
Cerebrovascular Surgery (2-3 years), Epilepsy Surgery (2-3 years), Interventional Neuroradiology (2 years), Neuro-oncology (1-2 years), Neurosurgical Critical Care (2 years), Neurotrauma (1-2 years), Pediatric Neurological Surgery (2 years), Peripheral Nerve Surgery (1-2 years), Skull-base Surgery (1-2 years), Spine

Surgery (1-year), Stereotactic and Functional Neurosurgery (1-2 years), Neurosurgery Research (1-2 years)
Median Income: $230,000 per annum

OBSTETRICS and GYNECOLOGY
Delivery of primary medical and surgical maternal health care to women of all ages.
Length of Residency: 4 years
Fellowships (1 to 3 additional years of training):
Gynecological Oncology (3 years), Infertility/Reproductive Endocrinology (3 years), Maternal/Fetal Medicine (3 years), Urogynecology (2-3 years), Pelvic Surgery (2-3 years), OB/GYN Research (1-2 years)
Median Income: $200,000 per annum

OPHTHALMOLOGY
Structure, function, diagnosis, and treatment of the eye and visual system.
Length of Residency: 4 years
Fellowships (1 additional year of training):
Cataract Surgery, Glaucoma, Neuro-ophthalmology, Ocular Oncology and Pathology, Ophthalmic Plastic and Reconstructive Surgery, Ophthalmology Research, Pediatric Ophthalmology and Strabismus, Refractive Surgery, Retinal Surgery
Median Income: $185,000 per annum

OTOLARYNGOLOGY
Diagnosis and treatment of conditions affecting the ears, nose, throat, oropharynx, and neck in patients of all ages.
Length of Residency: 5 to 6 years
Fellowships (1 to 2 additional years of training):
Otology Neurotology (2 years), Pediatric Otolaryngology (2 years), Otolaryngology Research (1-2 years), Head and Neck

Oncologic Surgery (2-3 years), Facial Plastic and Reconstructive Surgery (1-2 years), Laryngology (2 years)
Median Income: $210,000 per annum

ORTHOPEDIC SURGERY

Providing patients with the medical and surgical management of congenital, degenerative, and traumatic musculoskeletal conditions.
Length of Residency: 5 years
Fellowships (1 additional year of training):
Musculoskeletal Trauma, Adult Reconstructive Orthopedics, Sports Medicine, Pediatric Orthopedics, Musculoskeletal Oncology, Spine Surgery, Hand and Upper Extremity Surgery, Foot and Ankle Surgery, Orthopedic Research
Median Income: $260,000 per annum

PATHOLOGY

Definitive determination of the etiology and pathophysiology of various medical conditions.
Length of Residency: 4 years
Fellowships (1 to 2 additional years of training):
Blood Banking/Transfusion (1 year), Cytopathology (1 year), Forensic Pathology (1 year), Hematology (Pathology) (1 year), Immunopathology (1-2 years), Medical Microbiology (1 year), Neuropathology (2 years), Pediatric Pathology (1 year), Pathology Research (1-2 years)
Median Income: $160,000 per annum

PEDIATRICS

Diagnosis and medical management of a various conditions affecting infants, children, and adolescents. Pediatricians also routinely provide infant and childhood immunizations as well as regular check-ups.
Length of Residency: 3 years

Fellowships (1 to 3 additional years of training):
> **Sports Medicine (1-year), Allergy and Immunology (2 years), Cardiology (3 years), Endocrinology (3 years), Gastroenterology (3 years), Hematology (2 years), Hematology and Oncology (3 years), Infectious Disease (3 years), Medical Genetics (2-4 years), Nephrology (3 years), Oncology (2 years), Pediatric Pulmonary Medicine (3 years), Rheumatology (3 years), Critical Care Medicine (3 years), Child Neurology (3 years), Neonatology (3 years), Adolescent Medicine (3 years), Pediatric Research (1-2 years)**

Median Income: $125,000 per annum

PHYSICAL MEDICINE and REHABILITATION

Diagnosing, evaluating and treating patients with limited function as a consequence of diseases, injuries, impairments and/or disabilities.

Length of Residency: 4 years

Fellowships (1 to 2 additional years of training):
> **Electrodiagnosis (1 year), Musculoskeletal Medicine (1 year), Neurorehabilitation (1 year), Spinal Cord Injury (1 year), Sports Medicine (1 year), Conditions of the Spine (1 year), Traumatic Brain Injury (1 year), One- and two-year Research Fellowships in Physical Medicine and Rehabilitation are also available.**

Median Income: NA

PSYCHIATRY

Diagnosis as well as behavioral and medical treatment of mental, emotional, behavioral, and neurological conditions in individuals of all ages.

Length of Residency: 4 years

Fellowships (1 to 2 additional years of training):
> **Drug Addiction Psychiatry (1 year), Forensic Psychiatry (1 year), Geriatric Psychiatry (1 year), Child and Adolescent Psychiatry (2 years), Consultation/Liaison Psychiatry (1 year), Psychiatry Research (1-2 years)**

Median Income: $130,000 per annum

RADIATION ONCOLOGY
Definitive and palliative treatment of malignancies using ionizing radiation.
Length of Residency: 5 years
Fellowships (1 additional year of training):
Pediatric Radiation Oncology, Head and Neck Oncology, Gynecologic Radiation Oncology, Brachytherapy, Stereotactic Radiosurgery, 3-D Radiation Treatment Planning, Radiation Oncology Research
Median Income: $220,000 per annum

UROLOGY
Diagnosis and treatment (conservative versus operative) of a variety of conditions affecting the genitourinary system.
Length of Residency: 5 to 6 years
Fellowships (1 to 2 additional years of training):
Pediatric Urology, Reconstructive Urology, Infertility, Urologic Oncology, Female Urology, Urodynamics, Urology Research
Median Income: $230,000 per annum

Sources:
Association of American Medical Colleges (AAMC)
American Board of Medical Specialties (ABMS)
Fellowship and Residency Electronic Interactive Database (FREIDA) Online (American Medical Association)
http://www.ama-assn.org/cgi-bin/freida/freida.cgi

Most medical students enter medical school with a particular specialty in mind, but almost all end up changing their minds several times before making a final decision. Applying for a residency program is quite similar to applying to college and medical school. One must submit applications, write another personal statement, obtain strong letters of recommendation, and interview for each position. Most medical students confirm residency choices around the beginning of the fourth year of medical school and may spend the rest of the year solidifying their preference by taking part in elective clerkships and away rotations at desired residency programs. An alternative to diving into a specialty residency program is a Transitional Year Residency, in which the internship year is performed at a particular program. During this year interns can finalize their specialty choices and apply for second-year residency positions around the country. A small percentage of students (approximately 10%) choose not to enter the residency match for a variety of reasons. Many enter research fields and obtain a Ph.D. in a particular field of interest, while others choose to leave medicine to pursue other interests.

For more information, contact:
American Board of Medical Specialties (ABMS)
(800) 776-2378
www.abms.org

THE PREMEDICAL YEARS

Knowledge is power.

—Hobbes, Leviathan

Classes

Premedical Requirements: The following is a list of courses required by almost all medical schools for admission. Please note that they resemble the courses needed before taking the Medical College Admission Test (MCAT).

Biology and lab	1 year
Inorganic (general) Chemistry and lab	1 year
Organic Chemistry and lab	1 year
Physics and lab	1 year
English	1 year

Along with the traditional classes, many schools are beginning to ask students to have taken courses in the following areas:

Zoology, Calculus, Humanities, Behavioral and Social Sciences

Courses That Will Help You During Medical School: Let's face it; medical school is going to be hard. Schools require the bare minimum courses needed for admission, but you have always done more than the required work. The courses listed in the previous section will get you into medical school, but the following will help you get through it. I know that you cannot take all of these classes. Instead, pick the ones that interest you the most and spread them out over your final two years of college.

Biochemistry*   Microbiology*
Embryology   Physiology*
Genetics*   Psychology
Histology   Statistics

* I highly recommend taking these classes before entering medical school.

Courses for the "Well-Rounded" Physician: Today almost all universities require students to take courses in a variety of areas to complement their concentrated studies. Their goal is to produce graduates with a "total education," and this is also what medical schools are looking for. According to Dr. Pellegrino, writing in the Journal of the American Medical Association, "The central act of medicine—making a clinical decision—is only part scientific. To make a right and good decision for a particular patient requires thinking more properly derived from the liberal arts and humanities." I agree with Dr. Pellegrino's assessment, but I see no problem with students majoring in whatever field they find appealing. The key is to fill the rest of your education with courses in a wide range of humanities, behavioral and social sciences. A well-read, well-rounded physician is what we all hope to become. The doctor-patient relationship is based upon communication and the ability to relate to patients from different walks of life. In striving to become the best person you can be, hopefully one day your patients will see you as a humanitarian as well as a physician. Here is a list of important non-science courses:

Anthropology   Literature
Art / Art History   Music
Business / Marketing   Philosophy
Economics   Political Science / Government
Foreign Languages   Psychology
History   Sociology
Linguistics   Specific Cultural Studies

Choosing a Major

There are many conflicting views on what major premedical students should have. Some feel that science majors are too ordinary and liberal arts students have a greater depth of knowledge. Others say that doctors are scientists and a science degree will serve them best. My advice is to choose a major you feel passionate about, a field that excites your intellect. After all, you are going to study this subject for four years, and you shouldn't take courses just because you think the medical schools will look favorably at them. In reality, medical schools don't care what your major is. The only requirement they have is that you take the premedical courses compulsory for admission.

Statistically, liberal arts majors have a better chance for admission than some science majors (in particular biology), but you must be aware that there are far more science majors that apply to medical school. Recent data indicates that of approximately 16,000 accepted applicants to allopathic schools, liberal arts students comprise about 2,400 and the rest are science majors. This does not mean you should not study non-science subjects. I just want to belie the notion that liberal arts students have an advantage over science students. You have not yet become a statistic and, therefore, should not let numbers govern your choices. The best thing you can do for yourself is to pick a major you love and get the best grades possible.

Grades

There is no way to get around it; grades are important. They are so important that getting good grades should be your top priority in college. Grade point average (GPA) is the most important factor for medical school admissions. Schools place this importance on grades because they provide a quick way to determine the strength of a student's academic background. GPA demonstrates your ability not only to perform well in classes, but also the amount of effort put into studying. There are a lot of intelligent people that go to college, but only the ones that work hard consistently produce high grades.

What kind of GPA do you need for medical school? Unfortunately, there is no concrete answer for this question. But you definitely need a GPA of 3.0 or higher. Statistically, less than 5 percent of students with C averages get into medical school. In fact, the closer to 3.5 you are, the better *(see Figures 3.1 and 3.2)*. The reason I stress the importance of grades is that most schools decide to offer interviews based upon a student's GPA and MCAT score. Some schools even use a formula based on these numbers to rank applicants. Subsequently, students with low grades will find it difficult to get interviews regardless of how much they wish to become a doctor.

Figure 3.1

Mean GPAs for Applicants

	Application Year									
	1992	1993	1994	1995	1996	1997	1998	1999	2000	2001
GPA SCIENCE	3.13	3.15	3.18	3.22	3.26	3.30	3.32	3.34	3.35	3.36
GPA NON-SCIENCE	3.39	3.40	3.40	3.43	3.46	3.50	3.52	3.55	3.56	3.58
GPA TOTAL	3.24	3.26	3.28	3.31	3.34	3.38	3.40	3.43	3.44	3.45

Source: AAMC Data Warehouse: Applicant Matriculant File. As of October 24, 2001.

Figure 3.2

Mean GPAs for Matriculants

	Application Year									
	1992	1993	1994	1995	1996	1997	1998	1999	2000	2001
GPA SCIENCE	3.38	3.41	3.43	3.47	3.50	3.52	3.52	3.53	3.54	3.54
GPA NON-SCIENCE	3.54	3.55	3.55	3.58	3.60	3.63	3.64	3.66	3.67	3.68
GPA TOTAL	3.45	3.47	3.48	3.52	3.54	3.56	3.57	3.59	3.60	3.60

Source: AAMC Data Warehouse: Applicant Matriculant File. As of October 24, 2001.

Most students start college with a positive outlook and attend every lecture and do all the required reading. They may even start study groups and hold review sessions before exams. But it is commonplace for students to start cutting corners and try to get away with as little preparation as possible. This is an easy trap to fall into as one becomes more and more accustomed to college life. But there is a heavy price to pay. Not only will you find yourself stressing out for exams, but your grades will suffer as well. You will eventually take more difficult courses that demand greater effort, and having done well in previous courses will be a tremendous asset. I know you are saying, "I'm not going to do this to myself." But just keep in mind that there will be nights when you don't want to study, or you put off writing a paper until the night before it's due.

Many students start college with a poor GPA. This is to be expected when attending a competitive school with many premedical students. I was one of those students who began my second year with a poor GPA. The good thing was I had only about 30 hours under my belt, and so increasing my GPA wasn't impossible. I worked hard the rest of the semesters and my GPA grew rapidly. One the other hand, most students find that there will be little change in their GPA after 90 hours of coursework. The key is to recognize your strengths and develop a strategy for consistently producing high grades. Students have found the following list helpful in having a good GPA.

Tips for Increasing GPA:

- Take basic courses at a community college (your GPA for medical school applications includes all courses taken at all colleges).

- Sign up for undergraduate research courses (these grades are almost always an A).

- Ask senior students who the easy professors are and sign up for their classes.

- For every semester you have to take a difficult class, balance it out with one easy class. We all have to take hard classes in college, whether we like it or not. What's the point in having all of your courses be difficult each semester?

- To increase your science GPA, take introductory courses, such as Astronomy 101 or Geology 101.

- Take courses with optional final exams and ones that allow students to drop the lowest exam grade.

- If your GPA is close to the next higher tenth of a point (such as 3.49), take a really easy class to bump it to the next level. For some reason the human mind sees a large difference between a 3.5 and a 3.49 GPA. I suppose it's the same reason an item sells for $0.99 instead of $1.00.

I must offer one *caveat* concerning this section. Grades should be your priority in college, but do not neglect your responsibility to become involved in non-academic activities. You have to show the admissions committee that you will enter medical school having attained a "complete" education. One of the best pieces of advice I got during college was to not let my classes get in the way of my education. I know there is a delicate balance between grades and activities, but you owe it to yourself to develop into a well-rounded person. A student with a high GPA that has nothing to talk about will find that medical schools will not be very receptive. Instead, you should strive to become a student with academic successes, but having learned much more in college than how to study. We all have the expectation that our doctors are able to relate to people from all walks of life and are well versed in politics, religion, the arts, current events, and more. Why should you offer anything less?

Extracurricular Activities

Every year there are stronger and better-prepared students applying for those coveted medical school spots. Almost everyone works hard in college and will work as hard as possible to earn good grades and take preparatory classes for the MCAT. What if you were on the admissions committee? In front of you are applications from thousands of students. First, you weed out the students with the weakest grades and MCAT scores. But you still have tons of applicants left. How do you decide who will make the cut? One way to separate the truly deserving from the general pool is to look at extracurricular activities and make note of how the student allocated his or her time outside of classes and the library.

Extracurricular activities encompass everything you did other than what was required of you. This includes any employment, volunteer work, research projects, leadership in academic organizations, community service, athletics, and even overseas travel. Much of this work will have to be balanced with a regular schedule of classes, but you can take advantage of winter and summer breaks to demonstrate a sincere motivation to become involved with the rest of the world. The following is a list of extracurricular activities most premedical students participate in:

- **Hospital Volunteer Work**
- **Research Projects** ✗

- **Employment**
- **Tutoring and Mentoring** ✓
- **Athletics**
- **Fraternities and Sororities**
- **Student Government**
- **Service Organizations**
- **Science Clubs**
- **Honor Societies**

What are admissions committees looking for? They want to produce excellent doctors. There is no one definition of what makes a good doctor, but there are a few characteristics that we expect from physicians. Certain words come to mind like caring, compassion, intelligence, altruism, and empathy.

Another key to impressing an admissions committee is demonstrating leadership abilities. For example, it is much more important to be an officer in an organization than just a member. Almost everyone volunteers at a hospital during college. Although it is important to have some clinical exposure, this is not very original. I would suggest that students supplement this with volunteering at locations such as an AIDS or hospice center, homeless shelters, nursing homes, a camp for burn victims, or any other facility where people help people. These sorts of activities will not only separate you from other candidates, but also demonstrate a sincere desire to help those in great need.

While many medical students have no research background, there are advantages of having performed some research. A person having joined a research group will certainly have an understanding of the scientific process and commitment to science. If you decide to do research, try to get a publication with your name on it. Having a paper serves as proof that you didn't just spend a summer washing dirty glassware.

The Medical College Admission Test (MCAT)

He is able who thinks he is able.
—The Buddha

The Medical College Admission Test (MCAT) is undoubtedly the toughest standardized test offered to undergraduate students. An applicant's MCAT score, grade point average, and interview are the most important factors considered by medical school admissions committees to offer acceptances. It is possibly the most important exam a physician takes. Why? If you fail to perform well on this test, there are no future tests to take. It is similar to qualifying heats for the Olympics. If you fail to qualify, there is no chance to compete for the gold. Speaking from experience, the MCAT is like running a marathon and the keys to doing well are preparation, practice, and repetition.

Most students have problems with taking the MCAT because they stress out about the exam and combine it with poor preparation, like not having the right preparation books, focusing on material that rarely shows up on the MCAT, not understanding the format, or they start studying too late.

There is no excuse for not studying for the MCAT. I know we've all heard the urban legend of the student who didn't study at all and got a 38. But for the rest of us, reviewing for 3 to 12 months is the norm. If you don't study, you might as well throw your admission chances out the window along with the billion hours of research and volunteering you did.

What is the MCAT?

The MCAT is a six-hour long, standardized, multiple-choice exam taken by all medical students applying to U.S. and Canadian medical and osteopathic schools. Podiatric, veterinary, and chiropractic schools may also require the MCAT. The exam is offered twice per year in April and August. According to the American Association of Medical Colleges (AAMC), the MCAT "assesses problem-solving, critical thinking, and writing skills in addition to the examinee's knowledge of science concepts and principles prerequisite to the study of medicine."

The MCAT consists of three multiple-choice sections, Verbal Reasoning, Physical Sciences and Biological Sciences, and two writing samples. Many believe the MCAT serves to weed out those students who do not score well on standardized exams. Remember, the United States Medical Licensing Exam (USMLE) is also a standardized exam. Many schools tend to follow the theory that students who do well on the MCAT have a better chance of passing the USMLE.

How Do I Register for the MCAT?

There are two ways to register for the MCAT. You can register online at www.aamc.org/mcat, or fill out the paper version. Using the online application is highly recommended and less expensive. Paper registration packets are made available in February of each exam year and can be obtained from your premedical office.

For more information, contact:
MCAT Program Office
P.O. Box 4056
Iowa City, IA 52243
(319) 337-1357

You must register for the MCAT at least five weeks before the exam date. If filling out the paper version, the packet is required to be postmarked by a date printed on the application. Late registration is offered, but an additional charge applies. The MCAT is expensive enough (currently $180), and there is no reason to be late for registration and having to pay about $50 extra to the AAMC. A common mistake made by applicants is having improper postage and not sending the packet by registered mail with a receipt. It only costs a couple of dollars more, but at least you will know the forms were received.

Included in the registration papers are surveys about your background and level of education. This data is subsequently used by the AAMC to compile statistics of MCAT examinees. These days the MCAT application also requires a recent photograph for attachment to a MCAT ID card. It will be mailed to you after your registration papers have been processed. Photos may be taken at most drug stores that take passport pictures, or you can do like me and just sit in one of those picture booths and put in $2.00.

Test taking sites will also be listed and you rank your choices from most preferred to least preferred. In order to get the site you want, apply as early as possible. You do not want to drive a long distance to take the daylong test. Try to take the MCAT where you are familiar with the location, such as the college you attend or a local school. If you do end up with a testing location that is new to you, make sure to visit the site a week before the exam so you know exactly how to get there.

Suggested Coursework for the MCAT

At a minimum you should have completed one year of biology with the corresponding lab course: one semester of cellular/molecular biology, and one semester of structure and functions of organisms. One year of inorganic chemistry and the laboratory are also required. I know that many of you will have received credit for these courses through advanced placement exams. If you learned the material the first time, it should come back to you when studying for the MCAT. So there should be no need to take them again in college. Move on and take some other courses to enhance your college experience. Organic chemistry and organic lab are required as well. Some people say that only the first semester of organic is necessary, but I feel that you should take the second semester before the MCAT. Nonetheless, medical schools require it for admission, and having taken it can only help you on the exam. Finally, one year of physics, non-calculus based, is required for the MCAT. Science majors will probably be required to take calculus-based physics for their degree requirements. But there is no need to take on an additional non-calculus based physics course. In fact, the non-calculus physics questions will seem much easier than what you have seen in your class.

You may be asking yourself, "Do I really need to take the labs for the MCAT?" My answer is a definite YES. The MCAT always has graphs and figures accompanying the passages, and you will be accustomed to answering such questions.

Almost all colleges as well as medical schools require students to take one year of English composition and expository writing. Although not required for the MCAT, I urge you to take these classes before the MCAT. If you think about it, you will need the coursework for your degree and medical school admissions, so why not take them before the MCAT? The verbal reasoning section is difficult enough, and you should have as much reading comprehension ability as possible to perform well on all of the sections.

Some of you may be thinking about taking upper-level science courses to get an edge over the other examinees. Extra courses can help but are certainly not crucial for MCAT success. You can take physiology/anatomy or biochemistry/physical chemistry, but the extra material you learn may confuse you on exam day, or you may lose sight of the basic concepts the MCAT stresses. Keep this advise in mind if you are a science major, but do not alter the sequence of courses you take.

The key concept tested by the MCAT is reading comprehension along with factual knowledge. It may not seem obvious now, but reading articles found in journals and magazines is the best form of MCAT preparation. Go to the library and read periodicals like *Time, Newsweek, The New*

England Journal of Medicine, The Journal of the American Medical Association (AMA), *The New Physician* (AMSA), and *The Sunday Comics* (just to keep your sanity). You will not only be helping your score on the verbal reasoning and writing section, but the science sections as well. By the time you apply for medical school, the idea of reading medical journals will be nothing new and may provide something to discuss during interviews. I know from experience that being able to cite articles in medical journals is extremely impressive to admissions committees.

Figure 4.1

Courses for the MCAT

Needed	Supplementary
1 Year Biology (cellular/molecular biology and orgasmic/evolutionary biology)	Biochemistry
	Human Physiology
1 Year Inorganic Chemistry	Physical Chemistry
1 Semester Organic Chemistry	2nd Semester Organic Chemistry
1 Year Non-Calculus Based Physics	Additional Mathematics and Physics

Before You Start Studying

Before diving into those review books, you have to understand what the MCAT is all about. You should learn everything about the subject matter tested, the format and the scoring of the exam. This information is provided by the AAMC and is absolutely crucial to have. The AAMC has published the MCAT Student Manual, which includes practice questions and scoring keys. Other must-haves are the MCAT Practice Tests II, III, IV, V, and VI. They also include answer keys and provide tables to convert your raw scores to scale scores. MCAT Practice Test VI is the latest exam released and even has an answer explanation booklet. Get these practice exams, set aside an entire day to take them, and pretend you were taking the real thing. These exams are probably the closest thing to the MCAT you will take, and they will help you understand the stamina needed.

Recently, the AAMC has announced the beginning of a MCAT Practice Online service providing Internet access to nearly 900 authentic MCAT items through four full-length MCAT Practice Tests: MCAT Practice Tests III, IV, V, and VI. Features include automated scoring, integrated solutions, customized item selection, and diagnostic reports to help target your studies. It may be cheaper to buy full access to the questions rather than purchasing the individual tests. For current information please visit: www.e-mcat.com.

April versus August: The Great Dilemma

The consensus is that students should take the MCAT in April of their junior year so schools will have your scores by the time you apply to medical school. If you do take the April exam, try to limit the number of course hours you take during the spring semester. You can always take an extra class during the summer session. The key advantage of taking the April MCAT is the ability to retake the exam in August, if you want to increase your score. You will also have the option to have your scores withheld when you register for the MCAT. This way only you will receive your scores. If you're happy with the scores, you will need to write a letter to the AAMC section for student services authorizing them to send your scores to the medical schools to which you have applied. The only problems with this option are giving up your six free medical school reports, and your scores may be delayed for up to two months.

The August MCAT is a good choice for students who want to have the entire summer to study. If you take the August exam, make studying your only priority. Try to avoid working or doing research that summer. The main disadvantage of taking the August MCAT is having a delay in your scores reported to medical schools. Many schools will not interview students unless they have a MCAT score on file. Withholding your exam scores should not be an option when taking the August exam.

What is the Format of the MCAT?

The MCAT is comprised of four major sections: physical sciences, verbal reasoning, writing samples, and biological sciences. With the exception of the writing samples, the questions are all multiple-choice with four answer choices. You have about 78 seconds per question and this should be plenty of time, provided you have taken many practice tests. You have a total of 60 minutes for the two essays.

Figure 4.2

MCAT Test Day Schedule

Registration and Seating Assignment (includes having thumbprint taken for security)	ca. 1 hour
PHYSICAL SCIENCES	77 questions in 100 minutes (ca. 77.9 seconds per question)
Break	10 minutes
VERBAL REASONING	65 questions in 85 minutes* (ca. 78.5 seconds per question)
Lunch	1 hour
WRITING SAMPLES	2 essays in 1 hour
Break	10 minutes
BIOLOGICAL SCIENCES	77 questions in 100 minutes (ca. 77.9 seconds per question)

Celebrate it's OVER!!!!!

*Starting in 2003 the MCAT Verbal Reasoning section will have five fewer questions and it will be possible to score a 14 or 15 according to the AAMC.

Verbal Reasoning

The verbal reasoning section is similar to the verbal section of the SAT and AP English exams, but the material is tougher (as should be the case since you have a few more years of experience now). The verbal section is made up of 8 to 11 passages, followed by 6 to 10 questions (*remember in*

2003 the VR section will have 5 fewer questions). Subject matter ranges from the humanities and social sciences to the natural sciences. Students have reported having passages about astronomy, English law, history, and sociology, all in one testing session. The goal is to read the passages, be able to analyze the content, and use the material to answer questions about them.

For liberal art majors this section should be pretty straightforward, but many science majors find the verbal reasoning section the hardest. I know it was for me. The problem is that you really can't study any specific information for this section, and there are no formulas to memorize. You can't even begin to guess what type of material will show up on your verbal MCAT. It all comes down to how much reading you have done in the past years, not months, prior to the MCAT and the analytical skills you should have acquired throughout life.

About one year before you take the exam, you should regularly read articles in news magazines, and it wouldn't hurt to read the newspaper once in a while. But don't despair. You can bring up your score by understanding the types of questions asked, and practice reading passages and answering questions about them. I bought a book specifically written for the MCAT verbal reasoning section and it helped quite a bit. If this is your Achilles, you might consider doing the same.

Physical Sciences

The questions in the physical sciences section are comprised of one-half physics and the other half inorganic chemistry (freshman chemistry). You should expect to see around 10 or 11 passages with information specific to a certain situation, such as natural phenomena or a science experiment. Combined with your specific knowledge of physics and inorganic chemistry, you will be expected to answer 5 to 10 questions per passage. Many passages also provide tables and graphs to analyze. You should also be ready for around

15 straight questions not pertaining to any passage. These 15 questions should be a relief after having done so much reading so far in the exam.

Your performance on the physical sciences section should be a direct reflection of how well you did in you physics and inorganic chemistry courses. If you didn't do well in these courses, you should spend more time reviewing for this section and KNOW the formulas by heart. If all else fails, you can always take the numbers provided and put them in an applicable formula.

Writing Sample

No one really knows how important the writing section is for the MCAT. In fact, hardly anyone knows what the scores even mean. They do not contribute to your numerical MCAT score and are reported in the form of a letter (J through T). I didn't sweat this section at all and I'm happy I didn't. Unless you are applying to the Ivys, no admissions committee is going to care about your writing section score, and most interviewers probably do not know how to tell a high score from a low one.

I have to tell you do not totally blow this section off, as it will serve as a nice change of pace during the exam day. You will have 30 minutes to write each essay in which a specific statement will be presented. You are expected to write a cohesive essay centered on the topic. The official instructions provided by the AAMC are *"Write a unified essay in which you perform the following tasks. Explain what the above statement means."* The first task will be to explain what the statement means. The second and third tasks will be specific to the statement and are given immediately below the statement. The key to doing well on this section is to write an essay that is clear and completes all three tasks.

Biological Sciences

The biological sciences section of the MCAT tests your knowledge and interpretation of biology and organic chemistry. About 62 to 77 questions will be based on 10 to 11 passages, followed by 5 to 10 questions to answer. The passages may contain graphs and figures to analyze, just as is the case with the physical sciences section. The biological sciences also have around 15 straight questions, not passage based. The key difference between the two science sections lies in the fact that the biology and organic chemistry questions are not equally divided. You can expect to see around 65% biology and 35% organic chemistry, but these percentages have been known to vary test to test. *According to the AAMC in 2003, a few organic chemistry questions will be replaced by questions on DNA and genetics.* Again, this section should also be a direct representation of how well you did in biology and organic chemistry.

How is the MCAT Scored?

The verbal reasoning, physical sciences, and biological sciences are scored on a scale of 1 to 15. The AAMC takes the number of questions you got right, or the raw score, and converts it to a scaled number. A letter grade of J through T will be given for the writing section of the MCAT (J being the lowest grade and T being the highest).

Remember when you took the SAT and points were deducted for the number of questions you got wrong? Well, this isn't the case with the MCAT. You are in no way penalized for guessing on the MCAT and you should answer every question. Fill in every question blank on the answer sheet. If you don't know the answer to a question, go ahead and guess. Remember, there are only four answer choices. You still have a 1 in 4 chance of getting the question right. Hopefully, you will be able to eliminate at least one or two of the answer choices, thereby increasing your chances of getting the right answer. Trust me; the questions that you are able to guess correctly start to add up in your favor.

The AAMC converts your raw score to a scaled score by using a standard distribution (they curve the exam). The mean will be set around "8" with a standard deviation of about "2.5" for these three sections. This basically evens things out for the exam takers and takes into account that some questions were too hard. The conversion tables will be different for each exam administered.

You should also be aware that each time the MCAT is given, there are many different versions of the exam given. Subsequently, the test questions you have will be different from those sitting around you. This is done to prevent any sort of misconduct while taking the exam. You may be thinking, "What if my version of the MCAT had tougher questions than the person sitting next to me?" Don't worry. The AAMC uses a separate score distribution for each version of the exam given. You will be compared only to the people taking the exact version that you took. The AAMC can do this because of the large number of students sitting for the exam.

Figure 4.3

Mean MCAT Scores* for Applicants

Application Year

	1992	1993	1994	1995	1996	1997	1998	1999	2000	2001
MCAT VERBAL REASONING	8.3	8.3	8.3	8.5	8.5	8.6	8.6	8.7	8.7	8.6
MCAT PHYSICAL SCIENCES	8.1	8.2	8.3	8.6	8.7	8.7	8.9	9.0	8.9	9.0
MCAT BIOLOGICAL SCIENCES	8.2	8.3	8.5	8.7	8.9	9.1	9.2	9.3	9.3	9.2
MCAT WRITTEN	O	O	O	O	O	O	O	P	P	P

*Reported numeric scores are means; Writing Sample scores are medians.
Source: AAMC Data Warehouse: Applicant Matriculant File. As of October 24, 2001.

Figure 4.4

Mean MCAT Scores* for Matriculants

Application Year

	1992	1993	1994	1995	1996	1997	1998	1999	2000	2001
MCAT VERBAL REASONING	9.2	9.4	9.4	9.5	9.6	9.6	9.5	9.5	9.5	9.5
MCAT PHYSICAL SCIENCES	9.2	9.3	9.4	9.7	9.8	9.8	9.9	10.0	10.0	10.0
MCAT BIOLOGICAL SCIENCES	9.3	9.5	9.6	9.8	10.0	10.1	10.2	10.2	10.2	10.1
MCAT WRITTEN	O	P	P	P	P	P	P	P	P	P

*Reported numeric scores are means; Writing Sample scores are medians.
Source: AAMC Data Warehouse: Applicant Matriculant File. As of October 24, 2001.

MCAT Study Timetable

Months Before: In the months prior to the test administration, register for the MCAT and purchase the AAMC practice materials and student manual. This is also the time to make sure you have taken all of the coursework required for the exam and to develop an organized study schedule. If you are going to take a commercial review course, make certain to apply early and have all fees paid.

By now you should purchase the latest editions of MCAT review books. You need to study seriously for the exam and think of taking it as preparing for a race. Build stamina by working through practice passages and answering as many sample questions as possible. The goal is to perform your best on exam day, because this is where you want a "peak" performance.

38 • Future M.D.

One Month Before: The last month is key to performing well on test day. You should review each subject thoroughly until you know the facts and formulas by heart. Next, take a full-length practice text every week under the same timed conditions of the real MCAT. Your goal is to build stamina for the daylong test and create a sense of confidence in your abilities. Continue to practice by taking sample passages, making sure to analyze your mistakes. Keep track of the topics you have the most trouble with and study them in detail.

One Week Before: The last week shouldn't be that difficult if you took practice tests and scored about what you want to score. The Saturday before the MCAT, take a full-length test under similar conditions to what you will face the next week. The rest of the days, try to go through practice passages and review the major concepts. Don't forget to establish a good sleep pattern, eat healthy, and exercise.

The Day Before the MCAT: If you've been studying hard for the past few months, don't worry! Try to review the large concepts tested and solidify what you know. At this point do not study any new material, as it may cause confusion and you might forget what you already know. That evening put down your books, relax, and set out the items needed for the next day: a few #2 pencils, your favorite pen, your admission ticket, your completed MCAT ID card and picture ID with signature, and a timer. Remind yourself that the MCAT tests your critical thinking ability, not reciting every single detail of information.

Afterwards: Relax. You just finished an exam that you stressed about for months. That evening, go out and have a good time with friends and don't think about your score. There is nothing you can do to change your results, and worrying about it won't help either. Just wait for the letter to come in 6 to 8 weeks and go forward from there.

How Did I Prepare for the MCAT?

I studied hard for premedical courses suggested for the exam and tried to earn an A or a B in all of them. I bought a lot of review books and saved up enough money to take a commercial review course. The course wasn't really worth all that money, but I would definitely recommend it for all applicants, unless you have a great deal of self-motivation and drive to prepare on your own. I, like many of you, are accustomed to a classroom environment where we don't learn the material unless we are forced to. The books provided by the review courses are priceless and tailor-made for the MCAT, focusing on exactly what shows up on the exam. For me, taking a practice MCAT every week was reassuring that I could survive the daylong exam. It relieved much of my anxiety.

I took the August MCAT between my sophomore and junior years and it was the right decision for ME. The timing was right, because I had taken all of my premedical requirements and just finished organic chemistry during the spring semester. In the back of my mind, I was aware that if I did not perform as well as needed that I could potentially take the exam again the following April and August, if necessary. Fortunately, I was satisfied with my score and did not have to take the exam again. This timetable is not recommended for everyone, and no one should take the MCAT until they know the time is right and they have completed all of the suggested coursework. No one should have to go through such a grueling experience more than once.

One week before the MCAT, I took a full practice exam and scored lower than I wanted to at that point. Instead of dwelling on this "practice" exam score, I tried to remain focused on reviewing the major concepts tested. On the morning of the MCAT, I woke up really early and went over these same concepts once more, and I told myself that I KNOW the material and I WILL do well. Once the exam started, I felt like I was taking another practice test, and to my surprise the MCAT wasn't stressful at all. If you're wondering, I scored exactly what I wanted to. To this day I am convinced that having confidence in your abilities and intelligence are paramount to getting the score you want.

THE APPLICATION PROCESS

If anything is sacred the human body is sacred.
—Walt Whitman (1819-1892)

Many premed students mistakenly believe that the MCAT is the make-it or break-it point for medical school admission. More important than your performance on the eight-hour marathon are your life experiences and your inclination for pursuing a career in medicine. The application process gives you the opportunity to project an image of yourself on paper. Each medical school will keep a file that usually contains a primary application, a secondary application, an up-to-date transcript, letters of evaluation, and a photograph.

Before discussing the contents of the application, it is important to note the timeframe for this process. An important piece of advice to keep in mind is to *finish everything as early as possible.* The reason behind this is simple. Medical schools start filling their coveted seats as soon as they can. At one particular medical school, the files are reviewed every two weeks and ranked. Every time the admissions committee meets, they will move some of the top-ranked files into the "Accept" box, and the rest will be pushed over to the next meeting. Therefore, the earlier your file is completed, the more chances you have of being accepted. Nevertheless, the quality of your application should not be sacrificed simply to turn in your application early. If you believe you can significantly improve your application, then continue to work on it. If you are content with what you have written and believe the application is a positive reflection of you, send it in as soon as possible.

Determining Which Schools Will Receive Application

So when does the application process begin? Before actually starting with the paperwork, you have to decide which medical schools appeal to you. You should begin researching medical schools at the beginning of the year prior to your entrance into medical school. The Internet provides a great starting place for your research. Additionally, each medical school has a published view book that can be mailed to you by contacting the admissions office.

There are many factors to consider when deciding how many schools will receive your application. First, ask yourself if you would actually attend the medical school if you gained admission. If you answer no, then do not even bother applying. It will be a waste of your time and money. In addition, you should determine if the school's strengths are similar to your interests. For example, you probably would not want to go to The University of Chicago Medical School if you were interested in pursuing a career in rural medicine. But you would definitely want to consider Johns Hopkins Medical School or Harvard Medical School if you were interested in leading-edge research. Simply put, apply to the schools you would consider attending. This requires doing your homework by looking into what each school has to offer.

Applying to medical school can be a very expensive endeavor. The primary application costs about $50 for each school. The secondary application can range between $45-$90 per application. If you are invited for an interview, you will also have to pay transportation costs and hotel expenses. Take this into consideration as you choose the number of applications that you will submit.

There is no guarantee that you will be accepted to medical school. It is a very competitive process that can surprise even a confident premed with a 42 MCAT with rejection letters. You should probably choose five or six schools where you have a good chance of getting in. Then, pick three dream schools that may be somewhat out of your reach. In contrast to college, there are no "safety" medical schools. The public state schools do give you a strong advantage, and in most cases you should always apply to them.

Since these schools selectively admit students from their own state, you should have a better chance of admission. The Association of American Medical Colleges (AAMC) publishes admission statistics available as the *Medical School Admissions Report (MSAR)*. This information can help you judge how selective the individual medical schools actually are. The MSAR also provides data for the number of in-state and out-of-state applicants who were admitted to each medical school. You should look at these numbers carefully if you are an out-of-state applicant, because many schools overwhelmingly restrict their admission population to in-state students.

The American Medical College Application Service (AMCAS)

After narrowing down your list of schools, you should take the first step in the actual application process: the primary application. For most allopathic medical schools, the primary application is the American Medical College Application Service (AMCAS) form. These applications and the schools *not* associated with the AMCAS application are discussed below.

American Medical College Application Service (AMCAS): The Association of American Medical Colleges (AAMC) processes all the AMCAS forms and distributes your application to the medical schools that you have indicated. The AAMC does not make any admissions decisions, but simply distributes your information to the appropriate medical schools. The application form has not changed significantly over the past few years. Therefore, you should familiarize yourself by obtaining the latest version of the application from the AAMC website at www.aamc.org. *Starting in 2002, the AMCAS application will be accessible only via the Internet.*

The entire application consists of only four pages, but do not let that deceive you, because those four pages require a lot of effort. The first section consists of providing your personal information (name, address, other) and listing the colleges you attended after high school. The next section allows you to list your post-secondary honors and awards. You should also include membership into any honor societies. You also have the opportunity to list any extracurricular activities, volunteering, and part- or full-time employment.

The open-ended essay question allows you to discuss any personal experiences that would help the admissions committee in its decision. The essay is formally known as the Personal Comments or the Personal Statement. You have one page (single-spaced, approximately 5300 characters) to write about anything you wish. Further advice about constructing this essay is found in the next chapter. You should devote a significant amount of time to prepare answers to these questions, because the admissions committee may read them closely.

The last section consists of listing all the courses you have taken during your college years. With an official copy of your transcript, this section should be finished easily. The AAMC will verify all your listed courses with your transcript, and any discrepancies will cause delays in your application. Also, you will need to list the medical schools where you want the applications sent. You should consult the instruction booklet or the AAMC website to determine how much money should be included.

AMCAS applications are made available around the start of May of the application year. You should submit your application as early as possible without sacrificing the quality of your work. Proper planning is essential because you will probably have other commitments. The deadline for the application depends on the medical school, but it is generally between October and December. *Starting with the entering class of 2002, the AMCAS application fee will be $130 for the first designated school and $30 for each additional school. Those unable to pay this fee may apply for a waiver through the AAMC Fee Assistance Program (FAP).*

After submitting your application, you need to verify that your file is complete. After your file has been created with the AAMC, you are able to check the status of your application through their website. Additionally, the AAMC will send a Transcript Status Report if any transcripts are missing after your application has been submitted. You will also receive a Transmittal Notification approximately 4 to 6 weeks after your file is complete. If you have any problems with your application materials, you should contact the AAMC through their website.

Non-AMCAS Schools

A handful of medical schools have separate applications not affiliated with the AAMC or any of the other central application services. These include the following:

- Brown University School of Medicine
- Columbia University College of Physicians and Surgeons
- New York University School of Medicine
- University of North Dakota School of Medicine
- University of Missouri—Kansas City School of Medicine

For each of these schools, you will need to contact the admissions office to request an application. The specific guidelines that you will have to follow will be detailed in the application materials. The completed applications should be sent back directly to the school, since they are not associated with the AAMC.

The following application services are associated with a number of non-AMCAS schools and have their own centralized applications:

- The American Association of Colleges of Osteopathic Medicine Application Service (AACOMAS)

- **Ontario Medical School Application Service (OMSAS):** McMaster University, University of Ottawa, Queen's University, University of Toronto, and The University of Western Ontario.

- **Texas Medical and Dental School Application Service (TMDSAS):** UT Southwestern at Dallas, UT Galveston, UT Houston, UT San Antonio, Texas A&M College of Medicine, Texas Tech College of Medicine, University of North Texas Health Science Center (UNTHSC)—College of Osteopathic Medicine (TCOM).

American Association of Colleges of Osteopathic Medicine Application Service (AACOMAS): The American Association of Colleges of Osteopathic Medicine (AACOM) provides a centralized application process through AACOM's Application Service AACOMAS. They will forward the applicant's information to the appropriate osteopathic schools designated. Students can file one application and a single set of official transcripts and MCAT scores. AACOMAS then verifies and distributes these to each of the colleges designated by the applicant. AACOMAS also uses an Internet application found at http://aacom.org/students/application.html.

For more information, contact:
AACOMAS
5550 Friendship Blvd., Suite 310
Chevy Chase, MD 20815
(301) 968-4190
e-mail: aacomas@aacom.org

The Ontario Medical School Application Service (OMSAS): This is a nonprofit centralized application service for applicants to the five Ontario medical schools: McMaster University, University of Ottawa, Queen's University, University of Toronto, and The University of Western Ontario.

Applicants to Ontario medical schools submit only one set of application materials and academic documents, regardless of the number of schools to which they are applying. Applicants are strongly encouraged to use the Computerized Ontario Medical Application (COMA) diskette to make application to the OMSAS. It is the preferred application method of the medical schools. If it is not possible for you to apply using the COMA diskette, please contact OMSAS.

Each of the five Ontario medical schools has its own admission requirements. Applicants should be aware of the variations in the admission requirements, and be sure they qualify for consideration before indicating that they wish OMSAS to forward their application to a particular university. OMSAS will process and forward applications to all requested medical schools regardless of the qualifications of the applicant.

Candidates are advised to contact the school of their choice regarding additional information on the admission of applicants and for information on the academic program.

For more information, contact:
Ontario Universities' Application Centre
P.O. Box 1328
Guelph ON N1H 7P4
(519) 823-1940
www.ouac.on.ca

Texas Medical and Dental School Application Service (TMDSAS): The Texas medical schools, excluding Baylor Medical College, have a common application through the Texas Medical and Dental Schools Application Service (TMDSAS). This process is very similar to AMCAS and distributes your applicant information to the Texas medical schools. The application requires completing an online form, submitting transcripts, recommendations, photographs, and the application fee. The status of your application file and further information can be found at their website: http://dpweb1.dp.utexas.edu/mdac/homepage.htm. Overall, you have to provide the same information as in the AMCAS form. The online form also requires you to write a personal statement. The actual essay information does ask for specific answers: *"In your own words, explain your motivation to seek a career in MEDICINE. Discuss your philosophy of the medical profession and indicate your goals relevant to the profession."* You are allowed a maximum of one page for your response.

For more information, contact:
Texas Medical and Dental Schools Application Service
702 Colorado, Suite 6.400
Austin, TX 78701
(512) 499-4785
http://dpweb1.dp.utexas.edu/mdac/

Early Decision Program

The Early Decision Program (EDP) is another way to apply to medical school. This route allows students to apply to medical school, and you will be notified of admission decision by October 1st. Around 91 medical schools participate in the EDP, but this program has a few restrictions. *You can only submit an application to one U.S. medical school and must attend only this school if offered a space. You must apply by August 1st for AMCAS schools and submit supplemental information by September 1st.* If you are not accepted under the Early Decision Program, your application will be placed in the regular applicant pool and you are eligible to apply to other medical schools.

The only reasons to choose the Early Decision Program are if you are sure you want to go to a particular medical school, and you are a highly qualified applicant *(GPA above 3.6, MCAT scores of at least 9 or 10 on each section, tremendous extracurricular activities, and great letters of evaluation).* I strongly encourage students to think long and hard before applying through EDP. When applying to medical school, you do not want to limit your options. It is extremely difficult to decide which school to apply to and know that this school is right for you. One of the best experiences I had while applying was comparing different medical schools through the interview process. The way I was treated at interviews and taking a look at the location were key factors in making my decision where to attend medical school. I know it is comforting to apply to only one school, but is saving money and time really worth giving up your right to choose which school you shall attend?

WICHE and WWAMI Programs

What if your home state has no medical school? Well, don't worry because both the WICHE and WWAMI programs allow certain students to attend out-of-state medical schools without paying extra tuition. All western medical schools, except the University of Washington, participate in the Western Interstate Commission for Higher Education (WICHE) Professional Student Exchange Program. After certification by their states, students from Montana and Wyoming can attend a participating school and pay in-state tuition at a public institution, or a reduced tuition at a private school. The student's home state then pays a support fee to the receiving school. Students must apply directly to the participating schools of their choice, where they are considered on the basis of that school's admission criteria.

For more information, contact:
Professional Student Exchange Program
Western Interstate Commission for Higher Education
P.O. Drawer 9752
Boulder, Colorado 80301-9752

The University of Washington serves as a medical school for the five states of Washington, Wyoming, Alaska, Montana, and Idaho (WWAMI). This program allows students from Alaska, Idaho, Montana, and Wyoming to be admitted to the University of Washington and still pay in-state tuition. The students from these five states attend the first year of medical school at participating schools in their home states. The curriculum at each school is the same as the one at the University of Washington School of Medicine, and all students take the remaining three years at the University of Washington School of Medicine in Seattle. The admissions process is handled through the University of Washington.

For more information, contact:
Director, WWAMI
University of Washington
School of Medicine, Box 356340
Seattle, Washington 98195-6340
(206) 543-7212
e-mail: askuwsom@u.washington.edu

Secondary Applications

After submitting your primary application, most schools will send you a secondary application. The contents of these applications can vary greatly. Some schools, such as University of Pennsylvania, simply want your signature and a photograph. The other end of the spectrum is Stanford University, which requires over ten essay questions. Even many of the non-AMCAS schools will send a supplementary application. The lengthy secondary applications are often used to weed out applicants because many do not even finish them. Therefore, the actual number of applicants may be lower than what is indicated on the MSAR. In addition, all secondary applications require a fee that can vary from $35 to $90.

Since the secondary applications often change from year to year, you cannot do much preparation beforehand. Many of the secondary applications are accessible through the Internet, where the school gives you a personalized login and password. The topics you will be asked about vary from each application. A few of the essay prompts are given below to give you an idea of what you will be facing soon.

- *"Describe a difficult moral or ethical situation that you have encountered and how you dealt with it. What personal strengths, values, and beliefs helped you deal with this challenge?"*

- *"Why would you like to attend this medical school? What aspects interest you about our medical education program?"*

- *"Describe and discuss two or three personal accomplishments or projects in which you take particular pride. It is appropriate for you to include in your discussion what you have learned about your capabilities **and** your limitations from having participated in these activities."*

• *"Write a brief autobiography."*

The essay topics will usually ask about your personal experiences that reflect qualities required to become a good physician. It allows you the opportunity to present yourself on paper in a positive light. Additionally, you should tailor your essay responses specifically for that medical school. For example, if you were interested in practicing medicine in a large city, then emphasize that New York University Medical School would give you the opportunity to learn in a fast-paced metropolitan environment. In other words, try to convince the reader that you would be a good fit with the school. In fact, many of the secondary applications will specifically ask you to explain why you have chosen to apply to that particular medical school. If you have done your research on the school, you should be able to answer that question immediately. If you cannot, then why are you wasting your time and money applying to that school?

The deadline for the secondary application is usually specified when you receive the form. Most schools ask you to submit it as soon as possible, while others give a specific deadline. Similar to the AMCAS application, the sooner you submit it, the better off you are. Again, do not rush through the application and make careless errors. The quality of your writing means much more than the submission date.

You should read all the information that is sent with the secondary application packet. The medical school may ask for further documentation or information. This would also be a good time to submit an updated transcript if any changes have been made. Furthermore, the medical school will provide you with brochures and catalogs about their medical campus and the specifics on their education program. This can be a very valuable resource when completing your application and when making your final decision. The medical school will also give you an address where you need to mail your letters of recommendations. This is discussed further in the next section.

Letters of Evaluation and Premedical Committees

Letters of evaluation help in revealing an outside perspective of your past performances and the qualities you possess for developing into a skillful physician. With this in mind, you should begin to consider the type of person you want representing you. Getting a letter from a professor who has gotten to know you will mean more to the medical school than an ordinary letter from a famous, big-name researcher. The key is to select people who can share specific details about your character and work.

If you are attending a college or university, you need to locate a pre-professional or a premedical office, if it exists. Most colleges now have a premedical committee in place that acts as the coordinating center for all your letters of recommendations. Each office has its own requirements that can range from simply submitting your recommendations to interviews and additional forms. You should make an appointment with your premedical counselor, if one exists, to understand the office's requirements. For example, at Johns Hopkins University premedical students must submit recommendations, write a few essays, compose a ten-page autobiography, and be interviewed by a professor on campus.

The premedical office usually makes copies of all your recommendations and sends them to the medical colleges of your choice. Many counselors will review your file and write a cover letter that usually summarizes the content of your file. This process makes it very convenient for the writers of your recommendations, because they only have to send a letter to one location. If your school does not provide these services, or if you have already graduated, you will need to ask your evaluator to send his or her letter to each of the schools receiving your application.

Who should you ask? Generally, most medical schools prefer that you have at least two recommendations from science professors and at least one from a non-science professor. Some good people to consider asking include any research professors you have worked for, professors where you got an A or an A-in their course, research mentors, supervisors from summer jobs, coaches of the sport you play, volunteer coordinators, special programs coordinators, or others. In short, you should choose the people you know who would write honestly and effectively about your qualities. Many courses have teaching assistants (TAs), which you may have closely interacted with instead of the professor. This can be a tricky situation. Medical schools do not put as much weight on letters written from TAs. If you have no other option, then you should at least have the professor cosign the letter. The number of recommendations should be between three to four. Medical schools have a very limited time to review your file, so more than three recommendations is usually not needed, unless specifically requested by the medical school or the premedical committee.

The recommendations are the only part of your application where you are not completely in control. In many cases, missing recommendations are the reason why a medical school file is delayed for review. Therefore, you should plan to ask your evaluators as soon as possible. Professors can get very busy with their own work, so you should give them plenty of time to complete the letter.

Asking a person to write an evaluation can become a very nervous situation. You should relax and not feel like you are inconveniencing a professor by asking him or her to write a letter. It is a part of their job, and they should be happy to do it. You need to schedule an appointment with the evaluator and discuss your future plans of pursuing a career in medicine. When requesting a strong letter of support, you should carefully watch the reaction. If you see any hesitation, then you should probably try to find someone else. Once you receive a positive response, however, you should provide a file to hand to the evaluator that contains more information about you. This file should include your personal statement, transcript, resume, publications, and any other articles or essays that could give insight into your life. A simple method to display all your qualifications and achievements is to provide a well-written curriculum vitae or resume *(see Appendix E for a sample curriculum vitae and tips on writing one)*. The evaluator can use this information to report a detailed description of your academic abilities and personality.

Most premedical committees also have a form that each evaluator needs to complete and mail with the letter. The form also asks if you would like to waive your rights to see the letter. In most cases, it is recommended to waive your rights so that the medical school will not think you had any input in writing the letter. If you are concerned about what a particular person may write about you, then you need to consider asking someone else. You should also provide a pre-addressed, stamped envelope to either the premedical committee, or the specific medical school to which you are applying. After they have submitted the letter of recommendation, a thank-you note can be sent to show your appreciation. Most professors are usually very interested in their students' futures, so you should keep them informed about your medical school decision.

It is your responsibility to follow up with your evaluators to ensure the letters were sent. If they were not, then you should respectfully remind your evaluators while emphasizing that the letter should be sent as soon as possible. Your recommendations are a critical part of your application, and you should not procrastinate in asking your professors.

Transcripts

The AAMC requests that one official sealed transcript be sent to their office to supplement your AMCAS application. The process for ordering transcripts varies, but they are usually available through the registrar's office. The "Transcript Request Form" found in the AMCAS application should be given to the registrars of all the colleges that you have attended. The transcripts must be sent directly by your college to be considered official. The AAMC begins accepting transcripts only after the application is made available for the coming application year. Before making your request, you should carefully look over your transcript for any errors or missing grades. Having a copy of your transcript will also help when you are filling out your AMCAS application. Submitting the transcript as early as possible will get your file started and expedite the process when sending your actual AMCAS application. If any changes are made to your transcript after submission, the revised transcript should be mailed with an explanation to all the medical schools to which you have applied. Remember that separate transcripts need to be mailed to the medical schools not associated with the AMCAS form. Finally, transcripts must be sent from *every* college you have attended. This includes community colleges and courses taken by correspondence.

Photographs

Most secondary applications require you to submit a photograph. The admissions committee uses the picture to remember your face when they are reviewing your file. The picture you submit should actually resemble how you look today, so your high school senior pictures will not work. You should be dressed in business attire, and a smile wouldn't hurt. Please review the information about attire in the *Interview* chapter if you are not sure what to wear. To ensure your picture is not misplaced, you need to write your name, address, phone number, and social security number on the back of each one. The picture should be a wallet-sized photograph of your face and shoulders.

Medical School Applicant Numbers

The number of medical school applicants fluctuates year to year. According to the *Journal of the American Medical Association,* 1996 reported the highest number of applicants at 46,968 for 16,904 seats. Since that time, applications have declined five consecutive years. Much like the economy, the applicant pool shrinks and swells in cycles. In 1989 the number of applicants hit rock bottom at 26,915 for 16,749 first-year seats. But much like a wave in the ocean, the numbers rose steadily during the early to mid 1990s, and now they are dropping again. Between 1999 and 2000, the numbers plummeted 3.5%, and the year 2001 saw another decrease of 6%.

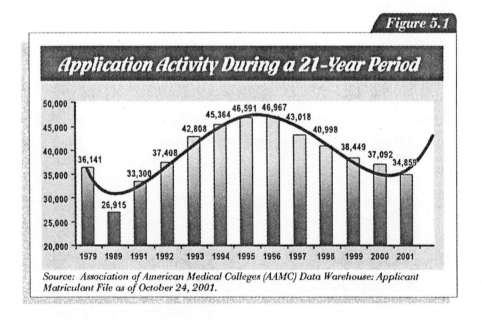

Figure 5.1

Application Activity During a 21-Year Period

Source: *Association of American Medical Colleges (AAMC) Data Warehouse: Applicant Matriculant File as of October 24, 2001.*

You might be asking yourself, "Why do the numbers change so much?" Simply put, it is the economy. When the job market is looking strong and students can get good paying jobs right out of college, some probably don't want to spend the many years required for medical school and a residency. As soon as jobs become scarce, medicine suddenly appears to be a safe investment. Everyone knows that doctors will have high paying jobs waiting for them when they finish school. This theory is widely accepted among admissions officers, but very few will admit that it is true. This also makes one wonder about the type of people who apply to medical school. You've probably wanted to become a physician for a long time and wouldn't dare let the stock market influence a career choice. But unfortunately, there are people in the world who do, and there is nothing you can do about it.

Even though the number of applicants changes, the quality of students offered admission does not. The mean MCAT scores and GPA tend to remain steady though the years. This essentially suggests that those students not applying to medical school during years experiencing declines were probably not good candidates in the first place.

How Many Schools Should I Apply To?

Most students send applications to around 11 to 12 schools. As stated previously, applying to medical school can become very expensive and secondary applications can be a pain to fill out. First, make sure to apply to all schools within your state of residence, because they offer the best chance for admission and generally the lowest tuition. If you have excellent credentials and good MCAT scores, you should consider applying to some out-of-state programs as well, but only if you truly want to go there.

It is true that your chances for admission are higher by applying to several schools, but this is only true if you are well qualified. Borderline applicants will find that the likelihood of an out-of-state, private school acceptance is very difficult. If you have difficultly getting into schools in your own state, the odds of gaining accepted to an out-of-state school are not promising. Also remember to apply to osteopathic schools, because many accept high numbers of out-of-state students. The only downfall of these private schools is the enormous tuition required to attend.

When applying to medical school there are very few absolutes. Thus, if you want to apply to 10, 20, or even 30 schools, by all means go for it. It's your career and you're the only person who knows what is best for you. Finally, most students judge their chances for admission based on the average GPA and MCAT scores of a given school. But keep one thing in mind: these numbers are only averages. That means that half of the students are above the mark and half below. Individual schools have a wide spectrum of GPA and MCAT scores with each incoming freshman class.

Final Thoughts on the Application Process

The most important advice is to try to finish everything early. In order to accomplish this, you need to make detailed plans and a timeline to keep you on track. There is a lot of paperwork associated with applying to medical school, and you will have to stay extremely organized. I suggest purchasing a file box where you can keep information about each of the medical schools. Even small things, such as a medical student's e-mail address, can eventually help you out when you are considering which medical school to attend. You should also keep copies of everything. Items sent through the mail can get lost and medical schools can misplace your application, so you definitely want to have backup copies. This also includes electronic files, because computers can mysteriously decide to delete your work when you least expect it. Staying organized will be one of the keys to a successful application process.

The application is your representative to the medical school, and you want to ensure you are viewed favorably. Feel free to practice filling out the application before actually submitting it. It is a good idea to have a friend carefully look over your application for any errors. Spelling mistakes are inexcusable and make you seem careless. If you have to submit the application on paper, type your answers neatly, showing that you are careful and complete.

During your application process, you will receive valuable information regarding each of the medical schools. While you are applying, remember to keep your eyes and ears open to any other advice or information you may come across. Your premedical office can be a great place to start, because they have the experience and staff to specifically deal with medical school applications.

Finally, remember that any contact you have with the medical school creates an impression of you. This includes your primary application, personal statement, secondary application, and your letters of recommendation. Your goal is to project the best impression that you can. The next step after applying is waiting to see if you have made a favorable impression on the medical school. If so, then you will have the chance for an interview to further assess your qualities. How you present yourself can make the difference between admission and rejection.

Partial contribution of this chapter was made by Chirayu J. Shah, Baylor College of Medicine.

ESSAYS AND PERSONAL STATEMENTS

My writing is simply a set of experiments in life-an endeavor to see what our thought and emotion may be capable of.
—George Eliot (1819-1880)

Basics of the Personal Statement

The personal statement will be part of every application submitted to medical schools. This is your chance to highlight personal achievements, accomplishments, and explain your motivations for becoming a physician. Medical schools are constantly looking for more diversified applicants entering into their programs, and you should use this opportunity to demonstrate your diversity and uniqueness. The applications themselves are not very different from one student to another, and a really well written personal statement can make one stand out above the rest. Your job is to convince the reader that you will add something special to the incoming freshman class. Subsequently, if you are an athlete or you climbed Mount Everest, tell them about it.

I strongly urge everyone to pour your heart and soul into writing what may be the most important statement of your life. Spend at least three months drafting the essay, and have it edited by an English professor and yourself at least three times. Grammatical errors could really make you look less than competent, regardless of your grades and MCAT scores. Another good idea is to have your premedical adviser review the final draft. They have seen thousands of essays, and it is easy for them to point out major and even minor pitfalls. Friends are also a good source of help, because they really know you and may remember things about you that you forgot to mention.

Before you start writing a personal statement, keep your audience in mind. According to the *Journal of the American Medical Association* (September 6, 2000), the overall ratio of men to women on admissions committees is 1.77:1. On average, 16% of committee members are from underrepresented minority groups. Although most committee members will be middle-aged, 74% of committees in the 2000 article had at least one medical student, with medical students comprising 15% of the total membership. Ninety-one percent of committees operate on a volunteer basis.

As you can guess by now, applicants should avoid making any sort of controversial statements, or placing too much emphasis on religious or political beliefs. Some students have found success with humorous personal statements, but unless you are really funny, I would avoid this route as well. If you are a relatively young applicant, be careful about stressing medical or life experiences. The admissions committee may think, "How much experience could a 21-year-old student have?"

The best time to start the personal statement is during spring break. You have the entire week to write down your thoughts and put them into essay form. By the time June 15th arrives, your personal statement will be ready to send in. The essay can be extremely crucial for borderline students. It can also show that, even though you may not have the best grades in the world, you will become a good doctor.

You want to catch the reader's attention early. The last thing they want to do is read another boring personal statement. A good idea is to start the essay with a life story that helped convince you to choose medicine. As you continue, list any specific experiences that have influenced your decision to enter medicine. The key item to remember is to be as clear as possible and to provide concrete details. Be sure to include any humanitarian/overseas work, clinical exposure, teaching or research experience, as well as any publications and oral presentations. Be careful, however, to avoid it sounding like a resume in prose form. Admissions committees love to see students who take on responsibilities within organizations and have leadership capabilities. If you have done so, include any changes or major influences you may have contributed by your involvement. Finally, describe how you wish to use your medical degree (academic medicine, rural medicine, political aspirations), and be able to describe why you want to take this path.

In reality, the likelihood that every member of the admissions committee will read your personal statement is small. They simply do not have the time to read the thousands of essays submitted. The only people who will read the statement will be your interviewers. After reading about you, the interviewer will gain more insight into your personality and ask probing questions about past experiences and accolades. Remember that all committees operate differently, and it is hard to gauge how they will operate from one year to another.

Instructions for Writing Personal Statements

What experiences, relationships, and aspirations have motivated you toward a career in medicine?

Comments must be limited to one page, no more than 58 lines. Comments should be no smaller than 10-point in size.

Sample Essays from Current Medical Students

(The names of applicants, institutions, and other items have been changed for anonymity.)

Example A

"Water, 2 shillings." The sign hung at an angle above a rusty faucet outside the old one room shack. "See that sign?" asked Dr. Ross. "Running water. These people are the lucky ones." As we wound our way through the narrow streets of one of Nairobi's slums, my host father began an impromptu lesson on daily life in Kenya. Dr. Ross revealed to me that about half of the slum's inhabitants were likely to be HIV positive—most unaware of their condition or its cause.

My experiences that first day in Nairobi, and throughout my three-month environmental studies program in Kenya, planted the seed that grew into my desire to become a doctor. What I saw opened my eyes to the tragic impacts extreme poverty can have on individual and community health. As I began my search for a fulfilling career, my mind often flashed back to the image of the slum. Though my path has been winding, my stay in Kenya, reinforced by later experiences with the inner city poor in the United States, began an evolution that ultimately led me toward medicine.

I graduated from New York University one year after my trip to Kenya, and hoping to use the problem-solving skills I had developed as a mathematics and computer science major, I began a job as a strategic consultant. Though I strengthened my analytic skills while researching industries and designing business models, I derived little emotional satisfaction from my job. I recalled the poverty Dr. Ross had shown me and began to realize that it was necessary for me to have a career in which I could help improve people's lives. After months of research and introspection, I concluded that medicine would best provide the intellectual stimulation to challenge me throughout my life, while enabling me to perform a vital service to society.

To confirm this growing sense that medicine would integrate service with problem solving, I began volunteering weekly at a health clinic for uninsured Latino patients. On one of my first nights at the clinic, I took the vital signs of a woman with advanced scleroderma. I listened intently as she explained her disease to me: the pain she felt as the skin around her jaw tightened, crushing her teeth together so that she could barely open her mouth. Our open discussion of her illness helped me empathize with her pain, and her gratitude for a sympathetic ear showed me the value of listening and caring. My interest in medicine solidified at the clinic as I talked with and provided "hands-on" help to patients, and as my curiosity about the human body grew.

After six months of volunteering, I left consulting to complete my pre-medical courses. My science classes emphasized the same critical thinking skills that math does, which strengthened my belief that medicine would complement my analytic skills.

Today, four years after my stay in Kenya, I am working with children at an inner-city boarding school, where I serve as a liaison between the residential and academic staffs. I started a volunteer tutoring program that exposes both volunteers and students to unknown worlds, as Dr. Ross did for me. At times I feel emotionally drained—consoling a 12-year-old who lost her father to a shooting death, or watching one of my favorite students meet the attorney appointed to replace his abusive mother and absent father. I have witnessed some of the socioeconomic challenges faced by my students, and I have realized that a patient's health must be treated holistically—by teaching children about the dangers of AIDS, encouraging individuals to change eating and exercise habits, and educating families about the importance of regular check-ups and preventative health measures. At the end of this school year, I will broaden my experience by researching Medicare at the American Medical Student Association, and will gain exposure to the medical policy environment.

My time in Kenya, at the clinic, in my courses, and at the school has confirmed my aspiration to provide medical services to people in need. I have experienced the fulfillment of making a positive impact on others, and I know that becoming a physician will allow me to make a greater contribution to society through public health. At the clinic recently, I translated a doctor's diagnosis of diabetes to a patient. Uncertain that he had understood me, I sat with the patient and his wife, scribbling the Spanish words for various foods under "Eat" and "Don't Eat" columns on a sheet of paper. Later, the patient's wife pulled me aside to explain her concern that her husband drank five beers a day. After verifying alcohol's effects on diabetics with the doctor, I quickly added "cerveza" to the bottom of the "Don't Eat" column. One month later, the patient and his wife returned. As they were leaving, she told me that her husband had not had a beer since his last visit to the clinic. She hugged me, whispering happily, "No mas cerveza, no mas cerveza."

Example B

I will never forget the first time one of my patients died. I was twenty-two years old, and somehow in the few short months since my college graduation, I ended up in a hospital room watching a man die. The day had started normally, consistent with my normal routine as a Patient Care Technician. I had spent the morning collecting vital signs, checking blood sugars, and helping my patients take their daily baths. Around eleven in the morning, we received word that we would be admitting a transfer patient from the ICU. He was thirty-three years old, on a ventilator, and dying of lung cancer. His fight had been long and hard, and his family was ready to honor his final request—he had asked never to by placed on a ventilator.

He arrived to his room around noon. The RN began her assessment as I took his vital signs. Though unable to speak due to the endotracheal tube, I understood clearly when he thanked me for bringing him an extra pillow. My attention then turned to the family, bringing them extra chairs and cups of coffee. I soon realized that although my help was greatly appreciated, there was nothing I could do to make their situation any better. And as he walked through the door, I realized the doctor was just as powerless. Three p.m. was chosen as the time that he would be extubated. In the interim, the hospice workers had arranged for a harpist to play in the room for him and his family. Before the harpist arrived, the patient's mother told me he would have much rather had Garth Brooks play for him, but the harpist would have to do. Next came the hospital chaplain, who prayed with the family. When the doctor arrived at three, the nurse and I entered the room and closed the door behind us. I was required to be in the room as the patient's tech, and was surprised to find that on some level I wanted to be there. I attributed this to my interest in medicine, but also realized that this was an experience I was bound to someday face. And experiencing what medicine was really like before attending medical school was the most important part of my job at the hospital.

After the pastor had led the family in a final prayer, the doctor removed the ventilator tubing. I stood by and handed pre-filled syringes to the nurse, who administered the stimulants at the doctor's request. The patient struggled to breathe on his own, while out of the corner of my eye I watched as the pulse oximeter reading plunged in to the forties. I realized it was time to turn the machine off. Ten minutes slowly passed. The patient's father stood over his son encouraging him to try to breathe, while his mother could only repeat, "We love you." Fifteen minutes passed and it was over. His labored breathing finally stopped, and the family was allowed to be alone in the room. It wasn't until I left the room that I realized that everyone had been crying: the nurse, the doctor, and even myself.

Later that day, I performed one of my duties as Patient Care Technician for the first time: morgue care. With the help of another technology, I removed his IV and Foley catheter, and labeled his body. We placed him in the shroud and called security to remove the body. A few minutes later I realized what I had just done. I went home knowing that I had experienced the end of one man's life. As someone planning to be a physician, this was an important step toward eventually practicing medicine and dealing with the patients that can no longer be helped. As a human being, it was one of the most poignant events of my life.

Example C

"No matter what happens, do not let go of her leg!" This was the way my first Saturday morning at University Hospital started. A call had come in that a van filled with children had been in an accident, and some had multiple injuries. At that moment, the ER needed as much help as possible, and I was assigned to Trauma Room 4 with Rose, a frightened four-year-old girl. Fortunately, she was conscious but had an injured femur along with a head injury, and I was to keep her leg straight. I must have stood there for over an hour watching the physicians do everything possible to make sure she was stable. While relieved that Rose was going to recover, there was no way of knowing the extent of her suffering and emotional trauma. I wished that we could have done more for a patient in her condition, especially one only four years old. So I decided to stay until Rose stopped crying and was with her parents. Walking home that evening, I began questioning whether or not I wanted to pursue a career working in such a harsh environment.

Why did I question a career choice that I was certain of for so long? Conceivably it was because none of my previous experiences could have prepared me for what I saw that morning. Was it that I did not find medicine intriguing? Was it that I felt uncomfortable working in a hospital? My first exposure to medicine came when I spent Saturday mornings observing my father, a clinical microbiologist, peering into his microscope. I saw how diagnoses were dependent not only upon textbook knowledge, but also experience and intuition. This time spent in his lab showed me that individuals are enduring the effects of disease; they are not case numbers. This partially explains why I wish to combine clinical research and patient care.

While spending time in my father's lab provided a good background, my interest in medicine is also due to a lifelong passion for science. From the basic courses to research in forensic toxicology, I tried to prepare myself for the rigors of medical school. Starting my second year at college, I joined the laboratory of Dr. James Witt to begin research in the chemistry department. Taking part in undergraduate research proved to be one of my best decisions in college, and it taught me the importance of research with a direct application to modern social dilemmas. With the aid of an undergraduate research fellowship, my biological studies were further applied to the human body. Currently, I am enrolled in an honors tutorial course.

While continuing my research, I tried to experience as much as possible in college, so I decided to become president of the American Biological

Society. This was another situation that helped me learn a great deal about my peers and myself. Through a mentoring program and elementary school science enrichment, where I demonstrated basic scientific principles to a first-grade class, I found that I liked teaching others. To confirm that teaching could be part of my career, I applied to become a teaching assistant for an organic chemistry course. This experience was invaluable and taught me that students need much more than practice and review sessions. More importantly, they needed reassurance.

My goal is to become a physician trained in all aspects of medicine, including research and teaching, which will help determine the specialty I ultimately choose. After three years of college, two years of research, and a Saturday morning with a four-year-old girl, I definitely know why I want to become a doctor. Medicine will offer a life filled with patients like Rose, each one offering a chance for personal growth for patient and physician. My belief is that the mission of medicine is the relief of human suffering.

THE INTERVIEW

An inquiring, analytical mind; an unquenchable thirst for new knowledge; and a heartfelt compassion for the ailing—these are prominent traits among the committed clinicians who have preserved the passion for medicine.

—Lois DeBakey, Ph.D.

Significance of the Interview

Making it to the interview stage in the admissions process is itself a big accomplishment. Most schools interview only 10% to 20 % of applicants, so the majority fails to get to this position. At this point the school has acknowledged that your grades and MCAT score have met their minimum standards. Now they need to put a face to that glowing application. When a school offers an interview, not only does this say they are interested, but that your chances of admission have increased many fold. When comparing the statistics of students accepted to students interviewed, one sees that the numbers are not nearly as formidable when comparing the ratio of students accepted to the total number of applicants.

When you think about it, why would a school go to the trouble of offering an interview if they were not interested in you? In addition, the interview process gives the applicant an equal chance to interview the medical school. You should ask yourself, "Would I be happy at this school? Do I like the city? Do I like the curriculum? Do the medical students at the school seem pleased with their education?"

In general, medical schools give two to three weeks' notice before the actual interview date. This gives plenty of time to arrange for travel and accommodations. If at all possible, plan to stay with a medical student. Many schools offer this to interviewees, and it gives the applicant a chance to ask questions specifically related to that school. About a week before the interview date, contact the school and make sure they know you are coming. The last thing you want is to show up on the wrong date!

How Should I Prepare for the Medical School Interviews?

Some people think that the interview is the hardest part of the application process, but others say it's the easiest. The disparity comes from the amount of preparation a candidate has done. Before interviewing with any school, practice interviewing techniques. Mock interviews with a premed advisor or counselor are a good way to practice. The advisor or counselor is a person who has done this many times, as has the real interviewer. Mock interviews will help you recognize both your strengths and weaknesses, as well as help eliminate anxiety.

Current medical school interviews are fairly relaxed. Most of my interviewers reassured me that they simply wanted to get to know me and that they were not out to grill me. In the past, medical school interviews were notoriously stressful. But the days of sitting on three-legged chairs are over (they used to do this to judge how applicants could keep their balance while answering tough questions). You should, however, be prepared for the "stress interview." I did have a couple of these, and they were not enjoyable.

Once you receive notice of an interview, learn everything you can about the school. Know what the school is famous for and what areas of research are being developed. The best thing to do is go to the school's web site and read everything that is relevant, including current events at the institution. Another suggestion is to talk to other applicants that have interviewed and ask them about their experiences.

You should definitely research current events in medicine and do some reading on medical ethics. Some schools are notorious for asking these sorts of questions, and some schools simply provide a list of questions to ask the student. During one of my interviews, I remember the interviewer held up a couple of pages of questions that were provided by the admissions committee. The topics ranged from recent movies I had seen to health care management.

The night before the interview, read over your application one more time and always re-read your personal statement. The essay will be the source of many questions asked of you. It is also a good idea to take a copy of your application and personal statement to the interview. I have heard of occasions when the interviewer hasn't had a chance to review your application beforehand, or parts of the application may be missing. If you have done research in the past, it looks extremely professional to bring a copy of any abstracts or publications you may have. This is something that can make you stand out and be remembered by the interviewer. Be sure you can answer questions about your research. You do not want the interviewer to think you spend your time just washing dishes instead of having a true impact on the research process.

Once you arrive at the school, a member of the admissions committee will greet you and you will meet all the other applicants; applicants from around the country, applicants with graduate degrees, and some may already have a medical career. But do not be intimidated by the others—they are just as anxious as you are. Typically, you will be given a packet of information about the school. Much of this will include how much grant money is received each year, what the school is noted for, and everything ranging from customized notepads to a map of the city. If you are lucky, this package will include the names of your interviewers and when and where you are to meet them. If you get the chance, go to the library and perform a quick online search of your interviewers and find out what their research interests are. This could provide something to talk about during your interview, and you may find some common interests. Most Ph.D.s and academic physicians love to talk about their research (just try not to fall asleep while they're talking!).

Interviews are typically scheduled for about an hour and will be conducted one-on-one. Some have been known to be as short as 30 minutes and others as long as 1-1/2 hours. But don't judge the success of your interview by its length. The interviewer may or may not have the full hour to interview you, or they may just be doing this as an obligation to the school. The rest of the day will be filled with activities, such as taking a tour of the library and teaching hospital, and having lunch with current medical students.

Whenever I asked people about the interview process and how I should act, they said, "Just be yourself." But this isn't really true. You should be yourself, but be your "very best" self. You're not exactly applying for a job at a fast-food joint. I know this may sound strange, but please don't forget good personal hygiene. Remember to brush your hair and teeth and be on your best behavior. I know you're thinking, "Of course I'm going to brush my teeth!" But you would be surprised at the people you meet at your interviews. Some of your colleagues will let their guard down and act like complete jackasses. Trust me, the reviewers are watching you every second you are there. In fact, at one of my interviews we were divided for lunch and seated with a doctor from the community. He asked each one of us how we were going to choose which medical school to go to. One student gave a typical answer about weighing his options and seeing what each school had to offer. When he turned to me, I said I would probably go to the first school that said YES! Well, it turned out that that community doctor was on the admissions committee, and before we left he turned to me and said, "I'll remember what you said tomorrow in our meeting." Well guess what! One week later I got accepted to that school and my life changed forever. Moral of the story: When you interview with a school, make them think that their school is the one you want to go to. There is NO substitute for enthusiasm. The last thing they want is to offer a position to someone who has no interest in their school.

What Should I wear?

Look as professional as possible, like an attorney ready to go court. My best advice is to buy a new suit even if you have an old one, because it may or may not fit anymore. While you're at it, go ahead and buy a pair of new shoes as well. Believe it or not, people do judge others by the way they look and the way they dress (even M.D.s and Ph.D.s). Another good idea is to purchase a nice attaché with a notepad to write on. Showing up with an old backpack wearing a $200 suit really doesn't make much sense, does it? A precautionary measure is to bring an extra shirt or blouse in case you have a spill. Can you imagine how embarrassing it would be to go into an interview with a big coffee stain? I know this sounds like a lot of money, but remember how much you're spending on application fees and plane tickets. Consider it an investment in your future.

A Note on Grooming

I know that sometimes we can get so entrenched in the application process that we forget the basics of interviewing. Something I was told to do was to dress as conservatively as possible and make sure to look the part. Grooming is important for any sort of interview, and I would advise every applicant to make sure his or her physical appearance is appropriate for a medical school interview. For men this includes getting a haircut, because long hair can be a sign of immaturity. But make sure to get a haircut around one week before the interview date, because that is when it looks the best. Women should make note of having their hair well managed or in a ponytail, and try to wear some make-up but not too much.

If you are worried about looking too young, wear glasses instead of contact lenses. Again, do not wear any unusual frames or sunglasses. I would also avoid large amounts of cologne or perfume. Avoid smoking or drinking a cup of coffee right before the interview. Your interviewer might be sensitive to the smell. If you are concerned about your breath, carry some mints. Think of the interview as a blind date.

What if I Don't Know the Answer to a Question?

This is bound to happen to all applicants. The interviewer may ask an obscure question just to see how you keep your composure; for example, "what is the capitol of Pakistan?" He knows you don't know the answer, but he just wants to see how you react. Most importantly, do not make up an answer. The best thing to do is to say you really are not sure.

What Should I Ask the Interviewer?

The interviewer will always stop and ask if you have any questions. You should definitely have at least five generic questions to ask and a few specific to the school. Asking questions demonstrates that you are interested in their school and would like to know more about it. On the other hand, if you don't have any questions, the interviewer may think that you could care less about them.

Sample Questions to Ask Interviewers:

- How would you rate the graduates of the school with those of others?
- What sorts of research opportunities exist at your school?
- How do you like being a faculty member at the school?

• Are students assigned a faculty or peer advisor?

• How do you like living in this city/town?

Feedback

Sometimes the interviewer will give some sort of idea as to how the interview went, but don't count on it. One way I got around this situation was by asking, "Would a person with my interests fit in at this school?" More often than not I got a pretty straightforward answer. Sometimes the interviewers may even tell you they would love to have you go to their school, and may even spend the entire interview trying to convince you. This is obviously a very good sign.

Recently, schools have begun sending out letters prior to the official acceptance date stating that the admissions committee was very impressed with your application and interview. There is some debate as to whether or not these are "pre-acceptance" letters, or just a way for you to think favorably of the school. Either way, this also is a good sign.

After the Interview

Many students like to send a thank you letter to the interviewer, but this is completely optional. If you are not used to writing thank you letters, don't do so. And trust me—don't think that this will get you into medical school. But if you do send a letter, be sure to have the correct spelling of the name and address of the interviewer, and send it right away!

Sample Medical School Interview Questions

- Why do you want to become a doctor?
- Tell me a little about yourself.
- Do you know which field of medicine you are interested in?
- Tell me about your experiences in the medical field.
- Which schools have you applied for?
- How are you going to decide which school you will attend?
- Where do you see your career in ten years?
- Where do you plan to practice medicine?
- Why did you apply to our program?
- What qualities do expect a physician to have?
- What will you do if you do not get into medical school?
- Do you like working with others?
- How would you handle a stressful situation?
- Tell me your stance on euthanasia.
- What was your major and why did you choose it?
- If there were something you could change about yourself, what would it be?
- Has there been anyone that influenced you career choice?
- How would you solve the health care crisis in America?
- Tell me about your extracurricular activities and your role in each organization.
- Describe your research activities and the extent of your involvement.
- Describe one of your research projects to me as an adult and to me as a child.
- What if you discovered that your research mentor was fixing data?
- What would you say to a patient who asked you to end his life?

- What was your favorite/least favorite subject in college? Why?
- Tell me what you do in your free time.
- In what types of settings do wish to practice (group, private, or public)?
- How would you tell a patient's family that their loved one is about to die?
- What was the lowest point in your life and how did you handle it?
- Do you have any hobbies and do you plan on continuing them in medical school?
- What is your greatest strength/weakness?
- Do you feel that physicians make too much money?
- Tell me your stance on abortion. *(Actually, it is illegal to ask this question.)*
- Have you ever considered a career other than medicine?
- How much experience do you have working with a physician or in a hospital?
- How would your friends describe your personality?
- What was the last movie that you saw? What was the last book that you read?
- What has been the most exiting point in your life?
- Why did you do so poorly your first year in college?
- Would you risk your life to help a patient?
- What would you do if you saw a fellow student cheating on an exam?
- Tell me your views on alternative/complementary medicine?
- Do you feel that America as a whole spends too much money on healthcare?
- Would you be willing to give up an organ to go to medical school?
- How would you reform the American healthcare system?
- Can you tell me what a PPO/HMO/DRG is?

- Would you wish to become a doctor if they only made $30,000 per year?
- Medical school applications are on the rise/decline. Why?
- Are you interested in performing research while in medical school?
- What are your parent's occupations and have they influenced your desire to enter medicine?
- Have you always put forth your full effort in every situation?
- If you were to be an inanimate object, what would it be and why?
- Do you have any questions for me?

How Should I Answer Medical School Interview Questions?

You should think of the interview as a commercial for yourself and sell the idea that you have the ability to become a fine physician. This is difficult but certainly not impossible. Within that one-hour session, you must demonstrate exactly what you expect to receive from a career in medicine, and what you can add to the medical school class and the profession. During this small window of opportunity, you must show enthusiasm for medicine and treating patients, compassion, and the will to work hard for the rest of your life.

When answering questions about your accomplishments, be humble. If asked, "Did you really start a new mentoring program on your campus?" You should say, "I was very fortunate to be able to do so, and it would not have been possible without the support of the faculty adviser and the other students." Acknowledge any and everyone who helped you along the way.

Age can be both a disadvantage and an asset to your application. If you are an older applicant, state how your experience has made you more open to other ideas, because maturity is essential for medical students. On the other hand, younger applicants can utilize their enthusiasm for medicine.

Undoubtedly you will be asked questions of an ethical nature. Answering these questions can be tough and you should explain your stance on the issue, but clarify that you can understand how others may feel differently. This is a sign of maturity and understanding. As a medical student and a physician, you will be in contact with colleagues and patients who come from diverse backgrounds. This shows the interviewer that you can work with others without any inherent biases.

Key Points To Remember

- Be confident but not arrogant.
- Show you are concerned about academic performance, but not like a gunner.
- Demonstrate compassion, but do not come across as overly sympathetic.
- Describe any medical or research experience you have, but do not exaggerate your role.
- Be courteous and respectful.
- Display your individuality, but don't make them think you're off the wall.
- Shy away from being too firm on political and ethical issues.
- Be as mature and professional as possible.

CHOOSING THE RIGHT MEDICAL SCHOOL

The physician needs a clear head and a kind heart; his work is arduous and complex, requiring the exercise of the very highest faculties of the mind, while constantly appealing to the emotions and higher feelings.
—Sir William Osler, M.D.

All medical schools are required to maintain high standards to be accredited by the Liaison Committee of Medical Education (LCME). Medical schools in the U.S. and Canada offer excellent educations and are regarded as being the best in the world. This goal of this chapter is to help you decide which medical school will best serve your needs.

Comparing different medical schools can be a laborious task and requires a great deal of investigation. In order to start, you must know which factors differentiate one school from another. In some cases, schools may be right across the street from one another, but students may have totally unique educational experiences. Make sure to list features you find important when visiting a school, noting your first impressions of the students, faculty, teaching hospitals, campus, and overall environment.

School Characteristics

Location: A school's location can be one of the most important issues when deciding between two schools. Some are found in urban areas, others in rural. More often that not, students like to live in an environment they are used to. If you're lucky, you can attend a medical school located in the city of your choice. This can be the city where you grew up or where your family resides. Other students prefer to attend the medical school affiliated with their undergraduate institution. Also consider the climate of the city. Does it have harsh winters, extremely hot summers, or will it rain all year? Remember, you will be spending quite some time in this location and you should ask yourself, "Will I be happy living here for the next four years?"

Tuition: The determining factor for tuition will be your residency status and attending public versus private school. Typically, in-state residents pay much less than s at public schools, while private schools charge the same for all students. You have to find out whether or not a school will provide scholarships for out-of-state students and how much financial aid each school is willing to offer.

Housing and Cost of Living: Moving to a new city can be stressful for anyone. It will be necessary to determine what kind of housing is available and how much it will cost. The school's location is also a determining factor, because staying near campus is preferable to a location too far away. Housing can range from sharing a cramped apartment with three roommates to renting a spacious home. The key is to find a place near campus that fits within your monthly budget. I know of some schools that still have dorms and apartments for medical students only. The best source of information will come from current students and the school's housing division, if one is present. Finding suitable housing in a prime location should be done well before school starts in the fall to minimize relocation stress.

Each of us knows how expensive some cities are compared to others. A meal in one town may cost $25, but the same meal may only be $10 in another. The same goes for housing and utilities. Living costs differ greatly between certain cities, and you may end up saving thousands over the course of four years of medical school by making the right choice. Financial magazines publish yearly cost-of-living indexes, or you can research these online. While making that list of important features when visiting schools, also note the cost of items such as gas, meals, and rent.

Statement of Purpose: Each medical school publishes a statement spelling out its goals as an institution and the type of physician it hopes to graduate. Your responsibility is to read these objectives and decide if you have similar aims. Statements of purpose can vary slightly between schools, and they range from producing general practitioners to medical scientists. For example, Johns Hopkins University School of Medicine "fosters the training of medical practitioners, teachers, and biomedical scientists." Saint Louis University School of Medicine "strives to graduate physicians who manifest in their personal and professional lives a special appreciation for what may be called humanistic medicine." Each school has its own set of principles, and it is important to be aware of them, but keep in mind their goals may be different from your goals.

Source: Medical School Admission Requirements, 1990-2000, United States and Canada, AAMC

Funding: To assist with making curriculum changes, a number of medical schools receive funds from foundations. The W.G. Kellogg Foundation helps to develop programs in community based health systems. The Robert Wood Foundation aims at integrating basic and clinical sciences, and also offers grants to encourage students to become more interested in practicing general medicine.

Curriculum

Grading System: Medical schools have different procedures for measuring a student's academic performance. Traditionally, schools used the letter grade system for both the basic science and clinical years. In recent years more schools are beginning to offer pass/fail grading scales. Some medical programs evaluate students by the pass/fail system, but may also have "high" or "marginal" pass or "honors" designations. Some students prefer the familiarity of the letter grade system while others prefer pass/fail, because it can help eliminate competition between students. Most pre-medical students know the anxiety associated with having to make an A in all classes to keep a high GPA. A pass/fail system places emphasis on learning the material, not on grades.

Contemporary Courses: Medical schools are currently expanding curriculums to include special topics such as family violence/abuse, substance abuse, epidemiology, geriatrics, nutrition, palliative care, and prevention/health maintenance. Now the majority of programs requires courses on complementary (formally known as alternative) medicine or offers them as electives. In addition, some schools offer classes on herbal medicine, spirituality, acupuncture, homeopathy, meditation, and women's medicine. See if these types of classes are offered and how to sign up for them.

America is becoming more culturally diverse than ever. After starting clinical training, a lot of students realize the importance of understanding Spanish. I know hospitals have translators, but you'll be waiting hours before you see one. Communicating with Spanish speaking patients is no longer optional in some cities; it is a necessity. Find out if your school offers a class in Medical Spanish and, if so, when it is available.

Tutoring Services: Right now it may be hard to imagine needing extra help to pass courses. But medical school is much harder than any undergraduate education, and you may find yourself struggling with some classes in basic sciences. It is important to seek help when you need it, and most medical schools offer some sort of tutoring courses. You need to find out whether such programs exist, if they are free for all students, and the types of tutors available (teaching assistants, peers, professors).

Research Opportunities: By now you know the important relationship research has with medical science. Medical students often join research groups in basic sciences or clinical trials. Some schools offer fellowships for conducting research during the summer. If you are interested, ask if such programs are offered and how much they pay. Those students contemplating a career in medical research frequently choose to spend an extra year in medical school to take part in some variation of an "honors research or thesis." Also, see if there is an office designated specifically for medical students conducting research and the name of the director.

Early Patient Contact: What's the one reason we all want to go to medical school, to read heavy textbooks and take really hard exams? No. We want to see patients and learn how to treat illnesses. Find out the earliest you will learn how to conduct a history and physical (H&P) and write up progress notes about patients. Some schools will devote time during the first month of medical school to prepare students to see patients, while others won't let you near the hospital until the third year. Some schools will even assign students to a doctor in the community and offer preceptorships, where students spend time working under the supervision of physicians in their offices. These opportunities are a real bonus during the basic sciences years and may help remind you why you're in medical school in the first place.

Student Services

Student Health Services: You would think that medical students would have access to the best medical care at the lowest cost. But you would be surprised to learn that many medical students have no health insurance. All good medical schools must provide some healthcare service for their medical students, and office visits should be free of charge. Ask the student services office what kinds of options are available and what services are given (immunizations, prescriptions, x-rays, lab tests, psychiatric counseling, needle stick policy). Some schools may even have healthcare for spouses and children for a set charge per academic semester or year.

Library and Computer Facilities: While interviewing at schools, there will surely be a tour of the medical library. I know they're boring, but you should stay awake for a few things, because you'll probably spend many hours there during the first two years. See how large the study areas are, how many journals are present, and if it is open 24 hours during finals

Computer based instruction and use of the Internet are becoming more and more prevalent in medical education. Many professors use e-mail to answer questions and make additions to class notes. Subsequently, many schools require students to have a computer at home. But all schools on campus should have computer labs with the latest software packages and free access to online medical journals.

Taped Lectures and Note Taking Services: What happens if you miss a lecture? How will you review the lectures for that day? These are questions you'll be asking soon after starting medical school. Many schools have audio and/or videotape lectures, so you may view them at your convenience. Another common feature is a note taking service to transcribe notes and make any additional comments to the syllabus. The notes are placed in your mailbox, e-mailed to you, or placed on the school's web site. Find out the charge for this service and whether or not it is run by students.

Community Service Programs: As a physician you will be expected to spend time performing community service, and medical school is an excellent place to get started on the path of charity work. Mentoring, student-run clinics, and health awareness events are a few of the many types of volunteer work opportunities available to medical students. I know taking time away from studying can be difficult, but participation in your community now establishes a pattern of charity service. Medical schools should provide information about any upcoming volunteer opportunities.

Quality of Graduates: A good measure of the success of a medical school's graduates is the rate of acceptance to desired residency programs. This information is readily available for all schools. You should pay particular attention to the percentage of applicants matching with their first and second choices. A good program should have around 80% to 90% of seniors matching with their first two desired residencies.

FINANCING YOUR MEDICAL SCHOOL EDUCATION

If you can count your money, you don't have a billion dollars.
—J. Paul Getty

Everyone knows that medical school is expensive, really expensive. Money can cause a lot of problems in life, but it should not interfere with your education. Medical students have a number of sources for financial aid available, and medical schools will never turn anyone away because of a lack of money. I am among thousands of medical students coming from middle-class families who receive full financial aid. The key to getting help is learning about the process and locating all resources for financial aid.

Unless your parents are independently wealthy or you win the lottery, odds are you'll have to apply for some form of financial aid. Approximately 84% of medical students borrow money to pay for medical school tuition, books, equipment, and living expenses. For many of you, this may be the first time you have had to borrow money. But guess what? It probably won't be the last time. Hardly anyone pays for a car with cash, and I do not know anyone that purchased a house without getting a loan. Fortunately, there are some excellent loan programs for medical students. Most are low interest with repayment schedules generally spanning 10 years. This should be more than enough time to become established as a successful physician.

The Costs

According to the AAMC, the average tuition and fees in 1998 for public medical schools were $10,324 for in-state residents and $23,052 for nonresidents. The same survey reported private school costs to be around

$27,000 per year. Don't forget that you still have to pay for books, equipment, housing, utilities, insurance, and transportation. A survey of the graduating medical students in the year 2000 found the average medical school debt to be approximately $90,000. I know this sounds like a lot of money, but it's not as bad as you think. With the right kinds of loans and repayment plans, you shouldn't lose any sleep over paying the money back.

Applying for Financial Aid

The first thing every student has to do is complete the Free Student Application for Student Aid (FAFSA). Get used to saying this word, FAFSA, because it's extremely important for medical students. The application is available at your school's financial aid office, or you can call for a form at 1-800-801-0576. Now you can also submit the application electronically at the government's website: www.fafsa.ed.gov (the fastest way to apply). If you have received financial aid in the past, remember to fill out a Renewal FAFSA, just as you will each year in medical school. The deadline for applying is early July, but the government starts accepting applications on January 1st of every year. Fill out the FAFSA as early as possible. In order to do so, both you (spouse, if applicable) and your parents need to fill out tax returns quickly. A few weeks after submitting the FAFSA, you will be sent a Student Aid Report (SAR) confirming all your financial information and the schools you wish to apply to for financial aid. Check the accuracy of all data, sign, and return it quickly.

Federal Loan Programs

Primary Care Loan (PCL): The PCL is a loan given to medical students designed to increase the number of doctors in the primary care field.

Those who borrow must complete a residency in the following specialties: family practice, pediatrics, internal medicine, OB/GYN, or psychiatry. Students must also practice in their respective fields during the entire duration of loan repayment The government is really serious about the primary care residency, because the interest rate goes from 5% to 12% if you fail to comply with all of the requirements (be really sure you want to enter primary care before borrowing).

Federal Perkins Loan: The Perkins loan is one of the best loans provided by the federal government. The maximum amount allowed is $5,000 per year with an aggregate total of $30,000 (undergraduate and medical school). The best part about this loan is the 5% fixed interest rate and longer grace periods before repayment begins. The catch is only students in severe financial need are offered this type of loan. Thankfully, this includes many medical students.

Federal Stafford Loans: With Stafford loans the federal government provides low-interest loans that constitute the most common form of assistance for medical students. There are two types of Federal Stafford loans and they are both based upon financial need. Most students use a combination of the two.

> **Subsidized Federal Stafford Loans:** The government allows students to borrow up to $8,500 per year with a maximum of $65,500 total. The great part is that the government pays the interest on the loans while you are in school.
>
> **Unsubsidized Federal Stafford Loans:** Here the government allows medical students to borrow up to $30,000 per year with a maximum of $138,500. Here's the bad part. You are responsible for the interest while in school, and you have the option of making interest payments while in school or letting them accrue (paying interest on accrued interest). I strongly urge all students to pay the interest while in school, or you'll see exactly how fast interest compounds.

After doing some additional research, I found that not all Stafford loans are the same. Banks offer different incentives to borrow from their bank instead of another. For banks Stafford loans are virtually no-risk, because the government guarantees the loans, regardless of whether students default. Subsequently, banks will try to encourage students to borrow from them.

Those of you who have borrowed for college already know loans have "fees" attached to them. This means that when a student borrows $5,000, he actually receives whatever is left after the "origination" and "guarantee" fees are subtracted. They typically range from 1% to 3%, but some banks waive some of the fees, give them back after some time, or they may reduce the interest rates for making payments on time. I suggest researching different banks to find out what incentives are offered that can save hundreds of dollars.

Figure 9.1

Federal Loan Programs for Medical Students

Characteristics	Primary Care Loan	Federal Perkins	Federal Subsidized Stafford	Federal Unsubsidized Stafford
LENDER	Medical school financial aid office on behalf of the Department of Health and Human Services	Medical school financial aid office on behalf of the Federal Government	Bank or other lending institution, the Federal Government or an eligible institution	Bank or other lending institution, the Federal Government or an eligible institution
BASED ON FINANCIAL NEED	Yes	Yes	Yes	No
INTEREST RATE	5%	5%	Variable. Federal Government pays during school, grace and deferment; and 91-Day Treasury Bill plus 3.1% during repayment, capped at 8.25%	Variable. 91-day Treasury Bill plus 2.5% during school and 91-Day Treasury Bill plus 3.1% during repayment, capped at 8.25%
BORROWING LIMITS	Tuition plus $2,500	$5,000 per year; $30,000 aggregate for undergraduate and medical school	$8,500 per year; $65,500 aggregate for undergraduate and medical school	$30,000 per year; $138,500 aggregate for undergraduate and medical school
ORIGINATION FEE	None	None	3%	3%
GUARANTEE FEE	None	None	Variable	Variable
GRACE PERIOD	1 year after graduation	9 months after graduation	6 months after graduation	6 months after graduation

Alternative Loan Programs

Instead of borrowing exclusively from the federal government, some students opt for Alternative Loan Programs (APL) available from certain banks. These loans may be a better choice for some students, depending on the loan amount and repayment options. In some cases alternative loans offer lower interest rates, longer grace periods, and the chance to borrow more than your calculated financial need. Under these loans students, may end up paying higher "guarantee" and "origination" fees. Unlike federal loan programs, there is no cap on interest rates.

One of the most popular alternative loans is the AAMC MEDLOANS Program. The AAMC program offers many options for borrowing from government and/or private loan guarantees. MEDLOANS is noted to have competitive interest rates, flexible repayment plans, and interest rate reductions for prompt repayment. For more information on MEDLOANS, you can contact the financial aid office at your school, or call 1-800-858-5050.

Alternative loans are exactly that, alternatives. Most financial aid advisors say the best loans are the Perkins and Subsidized Stafford. The federal government pays the interest while in school, but they may pay only part of the costs. The next best options are the Unsubsidized Stafford and/or Alternative Loans. You should research the two types of loans and find the best deals.

Service Commitment Scholarships

The U.S. Armed Forces Health Professions Scholarship Program: Medical students can obtain help though the U.S. Armed Forces Health Professions Scholarship Program. These "scholarships" aren't really financial aid. Instead, they are contracts to provide service for the Army, Navy, or the Air Force. Uncle Sam will pay for all of your educational expenses and provide a monthly stipend, but you must agree to serve one year in the military for each year of support after graduating. Here's one more condition. Taking part in a residency program at a military facility does not count toward the service commitment. I know students who have agreed to serve, and they all say it's a great way to pay for medical school and not have the burden of repaying loans. For more information contact:

Air Force	Navy	Army
Headquarters, US Air Force Recruiting Service Medical Recruiting Division Randolph AFB, TX 78150 http://www.airforce.com	Commander, Navy Recruiting Command 4015 Wilson Boulevard Arlington, VA 22203-1991 http://nshs.med.navy.mil/hpsp	Headquarters Dept. of Army ATTN: SGPS-PDF 5109 Leesburg Pike Falls Church, VA 22041-3258 http://www.goarmy.com

Note: All Armed Forces Health Professions Scholarships require U.S. citizenship.

The National Health Service Corps (NHSC): The NHSC is administered by the Bureau of Health Care Delivery and Assistance in the Health Resources and Services Administration, an agency of the U.S. Public Health Service. The goal of the program is the improvement of primary care health services in health professional shortage areas (HPSA). The NHCS offers scholarships and loan repayment for selected students. In return, medical students must agree to practice in HPSA from two to four years.

For more information, contact:
National Health Service Corps Scholarship Program
Division of Scholarships and Loan Repayments
1010 Wayne Avenue, Suite 240
Silver Spring, MD 20910
(800) 221-9393
www.bphc.hrsa.gov/nhsc

Financial Aid for Disadvantaged Health Professions Students (FADHPS): The FADHPS is a federally funded program for students coming from disadvantaged backgrounds. The government awards up to $10,000 per year, depending upon the financial need of each qualified student. Following graduation, the student must enter a residency in one of the primary health fields within four years of graduating from medical school. After residency, the student must practice primary care medicine for at least five years.

Scholarships for Students of Exceptional Financial Need (EFN): The EFN scholarships are made available to students from low-income families. The federal government provides scholarship money to financial aid offices at medical schools, and the funds are distributed at their discretion. The scholarships cover tuition costs and all other expenses except for housing. Much like the FADHPS, students have to complete a primary care residency after graduating.

Figure 9.2

Federally Sponsored Service Commitment Programs

Characteristics	ENF Program	FADHPS	NHSC*
PROVIDER	Medical school financial aid office	Medical school financial aid office	Medical school financial aid office
BASED ON FINANCIAL NEED	Yes - including family resources	Yes - including family resources; student must come from a disadvantaged background	No
COMMITMENT REQUIREMENTS	Student must commit to a primary care specialty	Student must commit to a primary care specialty and practice for 5 years	Student must commit to a primary care specialty and practice through the repayment period
AMOUNT OF SUPPORT	Tuition and other educational expenses	Tuition and other educational expenses	Tuition, fees, books, supplies, equipment, and a monthly stipend

* NHSC requires U.S. citizenship

Other Sources of Financial Aid

Medical Student Research Fellowships: Research groups are always willing to take on eager medical students to work in their labs, even if it's only for a couple of months. If you're lucky, you might even get to publish a paper and/or receive credit hours with the help of a supportive mentor. Most research programs also pay well, and it beats waiting tables during the summer.

State Supported Funding: Another advantage of attending a school in your home state is eligibility for "state-sponsored" aid. Schools often require separate paperwork for state grants and scholarships. This "free money" is given away quickly and is a good incentive for filling out all financial aid forms early.

Merit Scholarships: Just like college, medical students can be awarded scholarships for excellent academic performance. The announcements should be posted near and around campus. The dean's office will have the applications forms.

Medical Scientist Training Programs (MD/PhD): Prospective students interested in medical research as careers should consider applying to MD/PhD programs (6 to 7 years of medical school combined with research). Many of the programs are funded by the National Institutes of Health (NIH) or by private endowments. Obtaining admission to an MD/PhD program is very competitive and requires students having done extensive research in college. In return, the candidates typically receive full scholarships and a yearly stipend averaging $20,000 per year, depending on the school. MD/PhD applicants are in a completely different applicant pool, and your commitment to research is the key to admission (*see Appendix B for a complete list of U.S. medical schools offering MD/PhD programs*).

Figure 9.3

AAMC Survey: Borrowing Sources of Graduating Medical Students

	1998	1999	2000
Federal Stafford Student Loan, Subsidized	78.5	79.6	77.8
Federal Stafford Student Loan, Unsubsidized	65.9	68.2	68.0
Federal Perkins Loans	32.4	35.5	33.1
Health Education Assistance Loan (HEAL)	17.3	16.6	5.4
Primary Care Loan (PCL)	5.2	5.0	4.9
Health Professions Student Loans (HPSL)	1.6	1.7	1.4
Loans for Disadvantaged Students (LDS)	1.7	1.6	1.0
MEDLOANS Alternative Loan Program (ALP)	19.5	21.1	18.8
Other Privately Insured Loan Programs	7.6	11.4	12.8
State Loan	2.6	3.3	3.4
University Loan	21.0	24.2	22.4
Other	6.3	9.5	8.8

Tax Breaks for Education

Lifetime Learning Credit for Medical Students: According to the U.S. Department of Education for those students beyond the first two years of college, or taking classes part-time to improve or upgrade their job skills, the family will receive a 20% tax credit for first $5,000 of tuition and fees through 2002, and for the first $10,000 thereafter. The credit is available for net tuition and fees paid (less grant aid) for post-secondary enrollment after June 30, 1998. The credit is available on a per-taxpayer (family) basis and is phased out as income levels increase.

Student Loan Interest Deduction: Allows an above-the-line deduction (the taxpayer does not need to itemize in order to benefit) for interest paid in the first 60 months of repayment on private or government-backed loans, post-secondary education and training expenses. The maximum deduction was $1,000 in 1998, $1,500 in 1999, $2,000 in 2000, and $2,500 in 2001. It is phased out for joint filers with incomes between $60,000 and $75,000, and to single filers with incomes between $40,000 and $55,000 (indexed after 2002). The deduction is available for loans made before or after enactment of this provision, but only to the extent that the loan is within the first 60 months of repayment. The loan amount eligible for the deduction is limited to post-secondary expenses for tuition, fees, books, equipment, and room and board.

Final Tips

- Fill out the FAFSA as early as possible.
- Check all of the information on your Student Aid Report (SAR).
- If you do decide to borrow, shop around for lenders and find the best deals.
- Keep track of all letters concerning your loans, scholarships, and grants.
- Minimize your expenses and invest wisely.

MEDICAL SCHOOL LIFE

I swear by Apollo the physician, by Aesculapius, and Health, and All-heal, and all the gods and goddesses, that according to my ability and my judgment, I will keep this Oath and this stipulation—to reckon him who taught me this Art equally dear to me as my parents, to share my substance with him, and relieve his necessities if required; to look upon his offspring in the same footing as my own brothers, and to teach them this Art, if they wish to learn it, without fee or stipulation; and that by precept, lecture, and every mode of instruction, I will impart a knowledge of the Art to my own sons, and of my teachers, and to disciples bound by a stipulation and oath according to the law of medicine, but to none others.

I will follow that system or regimen which, according to my ability and judgment, I consider for the benefit of my patients, and abstain from whatever is deleterious and mischievous.

I will give no deadly medicine to any one if asked, nor suggest any such counsel; and in like manner I will not give to a woman a pessary to produce abortion.

With purity and with holiness I will pass my life and practice my Art. I will not cut persons labouring under the stone, but will leave this to be done by men who are practitioners of this work. Into whatever houses I enter, I will go into them for the benefit of the sick, and will abstain from every voluntary act of mischief and corruption; and, further, from the seduction of females or males, of freemen and slaves Whatever, in connection with my professional service, or not in connection with it, I see or hear, in the life of men, which ought not to be spoken of abroad, I will not divulge, as reckoning that all such should be kept secret.

While I continue to keep this Oath unviolated, may it be granted to me
to enjoy life and the practice of the Art, respected by all men, in all times.
But should I trespass and violate this Oath, may the reverse be my lot.
                    —The Hippocratic Oath, 5th Century B.C.

A Medical Student's Description of the Basic Science Years

Ah, the first day of medical school, a day no doctor forgets. The morning is filled with an endless number of forms to complete followed by a series of immunizations. Then you are finally handed the prestigious white coat. You'll probably go home and wear it in front of the mirror just to see how you look in it. Guess what, you look like a medical student, a medical student who knows nothing about medicine. But that will soon change after receiving the list of courses to be taken the first semester. Next comes the customary trip to the medical school bookstore. I must warn you to get ready for some major sticker shock. Many students will also be expected to purchase their own set of medical equipment, and you may even go home and model your shiny new stethoscope as you did with your white coat.

What comes to mind when thinking of the first year of medical school? Anatomy lab, and that is one smell that will linger the entire year. The scent of formalin will permeate through not only your clothes, but also your home and car. Some students even notice the cadaver smell when eating. But you'll learn to get used to it; after all, it is a right of passage. Generally four students are assigned per body, and you will get to know these people well by the end of the year. Try to get along with them and work as a team, or your life may become very difficult.

Next come the lectures and the reading. At first you'll be shocked to learn how much studying must be done for each class everyday. But you did ask to be there and were willing to do anything to become a doctor, so just pour through the pages of text. After a while, you will be accustomed to reading a hundred pages or so per night, and you'll start retaining more and more of the information.

If all goes well the first year should pass quickly, and you'll be amazed at how much medicine you learned. At the end you will have established a study protocol that works for you, because each student has his own rituals to prepare for exams.

Between the first two years of medical school, most students get a little time off during the summer months. You can use this time doing anything at all. Some decide to join a research group in hopes of getting their name on a paper, and others prefer to work in a doctor's office. I spent this vacation time doing exactly that, vacationing. This will be the last real time away from school for most students, and you should do all of those things you always wanted to do but never had the time for.

At the dawn of the second year, one starts to repeat the following letters often: U S M L and E. Most students take Step 1 of the USMLE after the second year and much of the year will be spent preparing for the exam. Meanwhile, you will also be taking courses centered on pathology, pharmacology, and behavioral science. Most doctors confess that the second year of medical school is the hardest, because of the volume of material taught.

By the end of the first half of medical school, students should be very capable of obtaining a history from patients and perform a physical examination. Most schools have some sort of course designed to prepare students on interviewing patients. You should make a point of finding out which schools offer such instruction.

I must tell you that medical school will be a change from college, not only in the type of material taught, but also the environment in which you will learn. The first two years will make you feel like you're in high school again. You can't choose which classes to take or what time to attend them. Classes will begin at 8 or 9 a.m. and end around 3 or 4 p.m., with an hour for lunch. The same people will be in your classes everyday. There will be a tremendous amount of gossip and rumor about fellow classmates, and you may find yourself caught up in this mess. My suggestion is to stay clear of this and focus on coursework; your life will be less stressful. Finally, don't forget the friends you had before you came to medical school and stay in touch with your family. They can be a great source of comfort during these first two years.

A Resident's Narrative of the Clinical Years

(Contributed by Ajay V. Maker, M.D., Yale University School of Medicine)

I was rounding the corner in the hospital lobby when a classmate grabbed me by my white coat. "Doug says hi," she revealed. "I don't know what you did for him, but he and his wife talk about you every day…he said he may not have been able to make it through if it wasn't for you." I stopped, said thank you, and traversed my mind for "Doug." I remembered then. Mr. G (I never called him Doug) was a healthy Scottish man in his 30's with a thick red beard. He had presented with jaundice and was found to have obstructive carcinoma. I assisted in his procedure and rounded on him daily. "He lives next door to me," she continued, "I just wanted to say thanks."

…and that is when it hits you. Although you feel as if you are wearing a big sign saying, "BEWARE, medical student," with your short white coat and pockets stuffed with random physical exam tools and mnemonic cards, you are perceived as a physician by everyone you see in a medical context (and some in the community…I can't get my Italian barber to stop saying "Hey Doc" with a thick Sicilian accent every time I walk in!). Entering the wards is one of the most profound changes to occur in your career as a student and lifelong learner. Although on the surface it may appear as just another year in school, treating patients and working on a medical team affects your lifestyle, the way you think, the way you carry yourself, and even your cocktail conversation. There are times you may feel that you are being taken advantage of, not receiving any teaching, being sleep deprived, or even being ignored, but hearing about patients you helped care for, like Doug, delivering someone's child, seeing a patient you helped rehabilitate be discharged, humbles you and reminds one of the true privilege we have to learn medicine and to care for others.

What to Expect

The majority of medical schools spend the first two years concentrating on building a foundation in basic science knowledge, "drugs and bugs," and pathology/pathophysiology. Though more and more schools are introducing patient care and case-based learning into their education, you will still always remember the first day you step on the wards and round with the team as something completely new. More than likely, you will have just taken step I of the boards, and as such, will be the king of zebras (medical conditions rarely observed) and useless trivia for the team. It is possible you may never know that much basic medical science again in your life, but the wards are there to teach you how to file away that knowledge into the appropriate folders in your mind and to learn to think at the bedside, not in the classroom. Chances are that by now you have seen every possible pre-set background design that comes standard on PowerPoint, and seeing your patient relax after you sit with them during a nebulizer treatment will remain in your memory far longer than a slide of their FEV1/FVC tracing.

To be the perfect medical student on the wards is not difficult if you enjoy being there. As in any quest, the journey should be as enlightening and passionate as the goal, or perhaps another path may be necessary. Some basic pointers are good to remember.

Always arrive a few minutes early and be the last to leave. Most likely your team will not wait for you if you are late. Even if you have been there seeing patients since 4 in the morning, if you are late to rounds, it appears that you are disorganized. However, if you are there before them, even 30 seconds, it appears you have been there all morning.

Imagine that you are the patient and dress accordingly. Would a wrinkled, Betadine stained pair of scrubs under a white coat that is closer to beige than white inspire confidence in a patient? I remember having a bile stain on my white coat after pulling an NG tube, and the best I could do was to stick a piece of white paper tape over it twice a day. It was not a pleasant site.

Read about your patients in a good textbook and/or a review article. THEN go to the literature. Although you may appear a "smarty pants" quoting the latest clinical trial, when you have another patient with a variation on the disease and when it is time to take USMLE Step II, you will be happy to have read the basics.

Always feel comfortable with saying "I do not know" to your team and to your patients. Of course, follow up with "…but I will find out." No one will ever remember that you did not know a lab value or an answer to a question, but at this point everyone can recognize garbage. Be honest, never complain, and know the most about your patients.

Your responsibilities will be to participate in rounds, clinics, and teaching conferences. Your chief will let you know your call schedule and any other responsibilities you may have, such as presentations. You should be comfortable taking a history and doing a complete physical on your own. The most important skill to practice and learn on the wards is to give a complete, concise, and clear presentation of your patient from memory. Not only does this consolidate the patient for you in your mind, but it also conveys to the team and those evaluating you that you understand what is occurring in the patient and have the ability to communicate it. You will be surprised at how a good presentation can give you confidence, increase your rapidity of learning, enhance your patient care skills, and lead to more responsibility and freedom. Therefore, practice your presentations the night before. Call up a friend or sit with a classmate and try to give the history and physical (H&P) in less than a minute. The assessment and plan is a chance to try your intuition and display your knowledge. It is also your richest learning experience from your residents and attending physicians. The sharper your presentation, the more willing they will be to help you with the assessment and plan.

Timeline

Starting your third year, or after three semesters at some schools, you will have a set of required clerkships that you must complete to graduate. These include Medicine, OB/GYN, Pediatrics, Psychiatry, and Surgery. Your experiences will be based in inpatient and outpatient settings and will range from general medicine to subspecialties. Talk to your classmates and older students for selecting the best teaching services and schedules for your purposes. A little bit of advice: Unless you know that the attending is always around, do not choose a service based on the attending; rather, try to be with the best teaching chief resident and/or intern. Ultimately, they are the ones who will most directly affect your experience, and perhaps even your choice of a career.

If you haven't already done so, the period after your required clerkships is the time to decide what area of medicine you want to pursue, as you will cater the rest of your year to that goal. This is the time also to do appropriate sub-internships at your host institution and/or away, start thinking about your preference for who writes your letters of recommendation for residency (ideally, you thought about this while on that rotation), and find an advisor in your field of interest. This is a chance to do research time, if you are interested, especially if planning to enter into a competitive match, as it will help to distinguish you from the crowd. If research is your inclination, this is also an opportunity to take a year off from the wards and enter a lab and apply for fellowships. I have many friends who just wanted some time off and left the country for a few months. Still others took time to get another degree. Whatever you choose to do, make a schedule and stick to it. There are many resources, from your Dean of Student Affairs to your intern, who can help you make difficult decisions.

Your fourth year will be spent with sub-internships, USMLE Step II, interviews, electives, and possibly research. But the worst is over. This will be your time to read a book, go for a hike, spend time with your friends, and polish your medical skills. Revel in what you have accomplished and have fun.

A Final Note

Imagine standing on the corner of a street and watching a car coming in your direction. For blocks you watch it and anticipate its coming. Then it passes you in a split second and you see only its rear license plate. Rotating on the wards is a similar experience. Finally, after sitting in a lecture hall ad nauseam, you are in front of the car, doing what it is you came to medical school to do, experiencing what it means to be a healer… and then it passes you. Sure, there are times you feel as if the day will never end and all you want to do is go home and sleep, but my fondest memories of medical school, and some of my most profound experiences in life, were in that short time.

CONCLUSIONS

How did I get in? It's simple: by working hard and planning well. Having your act together by the time you apply to medical school is crucial, and this planning allowed me the choice of admission to three medical schools. I was lucky enough to choose my medical school and came to San Antonio because I prefer a large city and warm climate. Hopefully, you too will have such a luxury. This book should demonstrate exactly what is needed to get that acceptance letter.

I, like many of you, am a first generation American possessing a tremendous amount of respect for education. My parents came to America in 1972. They wanted a better life and wanted it here. Arriving with little money, they had one thing that no one could ever take away from them: Education. This thought was engrained in my mind and I continue to share it with others.

At the age of four, I started telling my relatives that I was going to become a doctor. Sure, they laughed, but I never gave up on my dream. All medical students probably have people in their lives telling them they cannot become a doctor. But if that were the case, every seat in medical school would be empty.

Good luck in all your future endeavors. You have earned it!

APPENDIX A: ACCREDITED U.S. MEDICAL SCHOOLS

ALABAMA
University of Alabama School of Medicine
University of Alabama at Birmingham
1813 6th Avenue, South
Birmingham, AL 35294-3293

http://www.uab.edu/uasom

E-mail	admissions@uasom.meis.uab.edu
Phone	(205) 934-2330
Fax	(205) 934-8724

- Public. Year Organized: 1859. Percent URM: 13; Percent Women: 37; Percent Out-of-State: 46; Mean Entering Age: 22; Estimated Annual Cost: Residents, $6,797; Nonresident, $20,391.

- Number of Applicants: 1,711; Number Matriculated: 165; Mean GPA: 3.59; Mean Science GPA: 3.5; Mean MCAT: (9.8 VR, 9.8 PS, 10.0 BS, N/A); Deadline: Nov. 1st

University of South Alabama College of Medicine
307 University Boulevard
Mobile, AL 36688

http://southmed.usouthal.edu

E-mail	lflagge@jaguar1.southal.edu
Phone	(334) 460-7176
Fax	(334) 460-6278

- Public. Year Organized: 1967. Percent URM: 9; Percent Women: 38; Percent Out-of-State: 5; Mean Entering Age: 24.5; Estimated Annual Cost: Residents, $7,000; Nonresidents $14,000.

- Number of Applicants: 1,128; Number Matriculated: 65; Mean GPA: 3.72; Mean Science GPA: 3.65; Mean MCAT: (10.0 VR, 10.0 PS, 10.0 BS, O); Deadline: Nov. 15th

ARIZONA
University of Arizona College of Medicine Arizona Health Sciences Center
1501 North Campbell Avenue
Tucson, AZ 85724

http://www.medicine.arizona.edu

E-mail	N/A
Phone	(520) 626-6214
Fax	(520) 626-4884

- Public. Year Organized: 1967. Percent URM: 15; Percent Women: 48; Percent Out-of-State: 0; Mean Entering Age: 23; Estimated Annual Cost: Residents, $8,800; Nonresidents, N/A.

- Number of Applicants: 608; Number Matriculated: 100; Mean GPA: 3.62; Mean Science GPA: 3.50; Mean MCAT: (9.5 VR, 9.5 PS, 9.5 BS, N/A); Deadline: Nov. 1st

ARKANSAS
University of Arkansas College of Medicine
4301 West Markham Street
Little Rock, AR 72205

http://www.uams.edu

E-mail	SouthTomG@exchange.uams.edu
Phone	(501) 686-5354
Fax	(501) 686-5873

• Public. Year Organized: 1879. Percent URM: 11; Percent Women: 35; Percent Out-of-State: 30; Mean Entering Age: N/A; Estimated Annual Cost: Residents, $8,520; Nonresidents, $17,004.

• Number of Applicants: 754; Number Matriculated: 147; Mean GPA: 3.6; Mean Science GPA: N/A; Mean MCAT: (9.4 VR, 8.9 PS, 9.4 BS, N/A); Deadline: Nov. 1st

CALIFORNIA
Keck School of Medicine at the University of Southern California
1975 Zonal Avenue, KAM 500
Los Angeles, CA 90033

http://www.usc.edu/schools/medicine

E-mail	medadmit@hsc.usc.edu
Phone	(213) 342-2552

Fax   N/A

- Private. Year Organized: 1885. Percent URM: 16; Percent Women: 43; Percent Out-of-State: 20; Mean Entering Age: 24; Estimated Annual Cost: $30,648 (all students).

- Number of Applicants: 6,174; Number Matriculated: 150; Mean GPA: 3.56; Mean Science GPA: N/A; Mean MCAT: (10.0 VR, 10.6 PS, 10.6 BS, N/A); Deadline: Nov. 1st

Loma Linda University School of Medicine
Loma Linda, CA 92350

http://www.llu.edu

E-mail   N/A
Phone   (909) 824-4467
Fax   (909) 824-4146

- Private. Year Organized: 1909. Percent URM: 6; Percent Women: 41; Percent Out-of-State: N/A; Mean Entering Age: 24; Estimated Annual Cost: $27,124 (all students).

- Number of Applicants: 3,990; Number Matriculated: 158; Mean GPA: 3.66; Mean Science GPA: 3.62; Mean MCAT: (9.5 VR, 9.5 PS, 9.5 BS, N/A); Deadline: Nov. 1st

Stanford University School of Medicine
300 Pasteur Drive

Alway Building M121
Stanford, CA 94305-5119

http://www.med.stanford.edu

E-mail   N/A
Phone   (650) 723-6861
Fax   (650) 725-4599

• Private. Year Organized: 1858. Percent URM: 12; Percent Women: 46; Percent Out-of-State: N/A; Mean Entering Age: N/A; Estimated Annual Cost: $27,735 (all students).

• Number of Applicants: 6,607; Number Matriculated: 87; Mean GPA: 3.7; Mean Science GPA: N/A; Mean MCAT: (10.0 VR, 11.0 PS, 11.0 BS, N/A); Deadline: Nov. 1st

University of California, Davis, School of Medicine ǂ
One Shields Avenue
Davis, CA 95616-8640

http://www-med.ucdavis.edu/

E-mail   medadmisinfo@ucdavis.edu
Phone   (530) 752-2717
Fax   (530) 752-2376

• Public. Year Organized: 1968. Percent URM: 12; Percent Women: 47; Percent Out-of-State: N/A; Mean Entering Age: 25; Estimated Annual Cost: Resident, $10,884; Nonresident, $20,268.

- Number of Applicants: 4,231; Number Matriculated: 93; Mean GPA: 3.60; Mean Science GPA: 3.60; Mean MCAT: (10.0 VR, 10.5 PS, 11.0 BS, P-Q); Deadline: Nov. 2nd

University of California, Irvine, College of Medicine ‡
Irvine, CA 92697-3950

http://www.com.uci.edu

E-mail   pharvey@uci.edu
Phone   (949) 824-5388
Fax   (949) 824-2485

- Public. Year Organized: 1896. Percent URM: 5; Percent Women: 44; Percent Out-of-State: N/A; Mean Entering Age: 25; Estimated Annual Cost: Resident, $10,630; Nonresident, $20,014.

- Number of Applicants: 3,931; Number Matriculated: 92; Mean GPA: 3.68; Mean Science GPA: 3.65; Mean MCAT: (9.49 VR, 10.78 PS, 11.01 BS, N/A); Deadline: Nov. 1st

University of California, Los Angeles, UCLA School of Medicine ‡
10833 Le Conte Avenue
Los Angeles, CA 90095

http://www.medsch.ucla.edu

E-mail   N/A

Phone (310) 825-6081
Fax   N/A

- Public. Year Organized: 1955. Percent URM: 30; Percent Women: 42; Percent Out-of-State: 15; Mean Entering Age: 22; Estimated Annual Cost: Residents, $10,630; Nonresident, $20,014.

- Number of Applicants: 5,244; Number Matriculated: 121; Mean GPA: 3.66; Mean Science GPA: 3.64; Mean MCAT: (N/A VR, N/A PS, N/A BS, N/A); Deadline: Oct. 1st

University of California, San Diego, School of Medicine
La Jolla, CA 92093

http://www.medicine.ucsd.edu

E-mail somadmission@ucsd.edu
Phone (619) 534-3880
Fax   (619) 534-5282

- Public. Year Organized: N/A. Percent URM: 30; Percent Women: 42; Percent Out-of-State: 2; Mean Entering Age: 23; Estimated Annual Cost: Residents, $10,324; Nonresidents, $19,708.

- Number of Applicants: 4,627; Number Matriculated: 122; Mean GPA: 3.74; Mean Science GPA: 3.70; Mean MCAT: (11.0 VR, 11.0 PS, 10.0 BS, N/A); Deadline: Nov. 1st

University of California, San Francisco, School of Medicine
513 Parnassus Avenue
San Francisco, CA 94143-0410

http://www.som.ucsf.edu

E-mail	N/A
Phone	(415) 476-4044
Fax	N/A

• Public. Year Organized: 1873. Percent URM: 20; Percent Women: 60; Percent Out-of-State: 2; Mean Entering Age: 23.5; Estimated Annual Cost: Residents, $9,940; Nonresidents, $18,924.

• Number of Applicants: 5,217; Number Matriculated: 141; Mean GPA: 3.75; Mean Science GPA: 3.75; Mean MCAT: (11.0 VR, 11.0 PS, 12.0 BS, Q); Deadline: Nov. 1st

COLORADO
University of Colorado Health Sciences Center School of Medicine
4200 East Ninth Avenue
Denver, CO 80262

http://www.uchsc.edu

E-mail	somadmin@uchsc.edu
Phone	(303) 315-7361
Fax	(303) 315-8494

- Public. Year Organized: 1883. Percent URM: 13; Percent Women: 46; Percent Out-of-State: 15; Mean Entering Age: 26; Estimated Annual Cost: Residents, $10,920; Nonresidents, $53,297.

- Number of Applicants: 2,398; Number Matriculated: 129; Mean GPA: 3.60; Mean Science GPA: 3.60; Mean MCAT: (10.0 VR, 9.9 PS, 9.9 BS, N/A); Deadline: Nov. 15th

CONNECTICUT
University of Connecticut School of Medicine
263 Farmington Avenue
Farmington, CT 06030

http://www.uchc.edu

E-mail   sanford@nso1.uchc.edu
Phone   (860) 679-4713
Fax   (860) 679-1282

- Public. Year Organized: 1968. Percent URM: 10; Percent Women: 50; Percent Out-of-State: 8; Mean Entering Age: 24; Estimated Annual Cost: Resident, $9,100; Nonresidents, $20,700.

- Number of Applicants: 2,220; Number Matriculated: 81; Mean GPA: 3.56; Mean Science GPA: 3.52; Mean MCAT: (10.0 VR, 10.0 PS, 10.0 BS, P); Deadline: Dec. 15th

Yale University School of Medicine ♦
333 Cedar Street

Post Office Box 208055
New Haven, CT 06520-8055

http://info.med.yale.edu/ysm

E-mail   medicalschool.admissions@quickmail.yale.edu
Phone   (203) 785-2643
Fax   (203) 785-3234

• Private. Year Organized: 1810. Percent URM: 18; Percent Women: 49; Percent Out-of-State: N/A; Mean Entering Age: 24; Estimated Annual Cost: $29,200 (all students).

• Number of Applicants: 3,093; Number Matriculated: 102; Mean GPA: 3.71; Mean Science GPA: 3.70; Mean MCAT: (10.68 VR, 11.78 PS, 11.64 BS, Q-R); Deadline: Oct. 15th

DISTRICT OF COLUMBIA
George Washington University School of Medicine and Health Sciences
2300 Eye Street, N.W.
Washington, DC 20037

http://www.gwumc.edu/edu/admis

E-mail   medadmit@gwis2.circ.gwu.edu
Phone   (202) 994-3506
Fax   N/A

- Private. Year Organized: 1825. Percent URM: 14; Percent Women: 50; Percent Out-of-State: N/A; Mean Entering Age: 23; Estimated Annual Cost: $31,800 (all students).

- Number of Applicants: 9,911; Number Matriculated: 152; Mean GPA: 3.53; Mean Science GPA: 3.50; Mean MCAT: (9 VR, 10.0 PS, 10.0 BS, P); Deadline: Dec. 1st

Georgetown University School of Medicine
3900 Reservoir Road, N.W.
Washington, DC 20007

http://www.dml.georgetown.edu/schmed

E-mail   N/A
Phone   (202) 687-1154
Fax   N/A

- Private. Year Organized: 1851. Percent URM: 26; Percent Women: 44; Percent Out-of-State: N/A; Mean Entering Age: N/A; Estimated Annual Cost: $28,650 (all students).

- Number of Applicants: 8,796; Number Matriculated: 171; Mean GPA: 3.59; Mean Science GPA: 3.56; Mean MCAT: (10.0 VR, 10.4 PS, 10.5 BS, N/A); Deadline: Nov. 1st

Howard University College of Medicine
520 W Street, N.W.
Washington, DC 20059

http://www.med.howard.edu

E-mail afinney@howard.edu
Phone (202) 806-6270
Fax (202) 806-7934

• Private. Year Organized: 1868. Percent URM: 60; Percent Women: 49; Percent Out-of-State: N/A; Mean Entering Age: N/A; Estimated Annual Cost: $16,460 (all students).

• Number of Applicants: 5,505; Number Matriculated: 113; Mean GPA: 3.14; Mean Science GPA: 3.02; Mean MCAT: (7.9 VR, 7.6 PS, 8.0 BS, N/A); Deadline: Dec. 15th

FLORIDA
University of Florida College of Medicine
Box 100215
J. Hillis Miller Health Center
Gainesville, FL 32610

http://www.med.ufl.edu

E-mail robyn@dean.med.usl.edu
Phone (352) 392-4569
Fax (352) 846-0622

• Public. Year Organized: 1956. Percent URM: 46; Percent Women: 46; Percent Out-of-State: 0; Mean Entering Age: 22; Estimated Annual Cost: Residents, $9,223; s, $26,033.

- Number of Applicants: 2,047; Number Matriculated: 115; Mean GPA: 3.67; Mean Science GPA: 3.72; Mean MCAT: (9.0 VR, 9.0 PS, 9.0 BS, N/A); Deadline: Dec. 1st

University of Miami School of Medicine
1600 N.W. 10th Avenue
Post Office Box 016099(R699)
Miami, FL 33101

http://www.med.miami.edu

E-mail   med.admissions@miami.edu
Phone   (305) 243-6791
Fax   (305) 243-6548

- Private. Year Organized: 1952. Percent URM: 10; Percent Women: 56; Percent Out-of-State: <1; Mean Entering Age: 24; Estimated Annual Cost: Residents, $25,670; s, $35,670.

- Number of Applicants: 2,410; Number Matriculated: 143; Mean GPA: 3.70; Mean Science GPA: 3.60; Mean MCAT: (10.0 VR, 9.7 PS, 10.3 BS, P); Deadline: Dec. 15th

University of South Florida College of Medicine
12901 Bruce B. Downs Boulevard
Box 2
Tampa, FL 33612-4799

http://www.med.usf.edu/med.html

E-mail	N/A
Phone	(813) 974-2229
Fax	(813) 974-4990

• Public. Year Organized: 1971. Percent URM: N/A; Percent Women: 30-35; Percent Out-of-State: <5; Mean Entering Age: 26; Estimated Annual Cost: Residents, $9,233; s, $26,033.

• Number of Applicants: 1,680; Number Matriculated: 96; Mean GPA: 3.60; Mean Science GPA: 3.80; Mean MCAT: (9.7 VR, 10.1 PS, 10.3 BS, N/A); Deadline: Dec. 1st

GEORGIA
Emory University School of Medicine
Woodruff Health Sciences Center
Administration Building
1440 Clifton Road, N.E.
Atlanta, GA 30322

http://www.emory.edu/WHSC

E-mail	medschadmiss@medadm.emory.edu
Phone	(404) 727-5660
Fax	(404) 727-0045

• Private. Year Organized: 1915. Percent URM: 30; Percent Women: 41; Percent Out-of-State: 50; Mean Entering Age: 23; Estimated Annual Cost: $25,770 (all students).

- Number of Applicants: 7,420; Number Matriculated: 111; Mean GPA: 3.69; Mean Science GPA: 3.70; Mean MCAT: (9.8 VR, 10.6 PS, 10.5 BS, P); Deadline: Oct. 15th

Medical College of Georgia School of Medicine
1120 Fifteenth Street
Augusta, GA 30912

http://www.mcg.edu

E-mail   sclmed.stdadmin@mail.mcg.edu
Phone   (706) 721-3186
Fax   (706) 721-0959

- Public. Year Organized: 1828. Percent URM: 5; Percent Women: 31; Percent Out-of-State: 5; Mean Entering Age: N/A; Estimated Annual Cost: Residents, $4,862; s, $19,448.

- Number of Applicants: 1,632; Number Matriculated: 180; Mean GPA: N/A; Mean Science GPA: N/A; Mean MCAT: (9.8 VR, 9.5 PS, 9.9 BS, N/A); Deadline: Nov. 1st

Mercer University School of Medicine
1550 College Street
Macon, GA 31207

http://www.mercer.edu

E-mail   kothanek.j@gain.mercer.edu
Phone   (912) 301-2524
Fax   (912) 301-2547

- Private. Year Organized: 1982. Percent URM: 4; Percent Women: 37; Percent Out-of-State: 0; Mean Entering Age: 24; Estimated Annual Cost: $21,144 (all students).

- Number of Applicants: 1,311; Number Matriculated: 54; Mean GPA: N/A; Mean Science GPA: N/A; Mean MCAT: (N/A VR, N/A PS, N/A BS, N/A); Deadline: Nov. 1st

Morehouse School of Medicine
720 Westview Drive, S.W.
Atlanta, GA 30310

http://www.msm.edu

E-mail   karen@msm.edu
Phone   (404) 752-1500
Fax   (404) 752-1512

- Private. Year Organized: 1978. Percent URM: 85; Percent Women: 55; Percent Out-of-State: 20; Mean Entering Age: 23; Estimated Annual Cost: $18,200 (all students).

- Number of Applicants: 2,982; Number Matriculated: 34; Mean GPA: 3.0; Mean Science GPA: N/A; Mean MCAT: (7.0 VR, 7.0 PS, 7.0 BS, N/A); Deadline: Dec. 1st

HAWAII
University of Hawaii John A. Burns School of Medicine
1960 East-West Road
Honolulu, HI 96822

http://medworld.biomed.hawaii.edu

E-mail   nishikim@jabsom.biomed.hawaii.edu
Phone   (808) 956-8300
Fax   (808) 956-9547

- Public. Year Organized: 1992. Percent URM: 15; Percent Women: 47; Percent Out-of-State: 11; Mean Entering Age: 24; Estimated Annual Cost: Residents, $10,824; s, $24,528.

- Number of Applicants: 1,098; Number Matriculated: 62; Mean GPA: 3.55; Mean Science GPA: 3.49; Mean MCAT: (9.00 VR, 9.47 PS, 9.90 BS, P); Deadline: Dec. 1st

ILLINOIS
Finch University of Health Sciences/ The Chicago Medical School
3333 Green Bay Road
North Chicago, IL 60064

http://www.finchcms.edu

E-mail   jonesk@mis.finchcms.edu
Phone   (847) 578-3204
Fax   (847) 578-3284

- Private. Year Organized: 1912. Percent URM: 12; Percent Women: 40; Percent Out-of-State: 63; Mean Entering Age: 25; Estimated Annual Cost: $32,270 (all students).

- Number of Applicants: 10,102; Number Matriculated: 104; Mean GPA: 3.23; Mean Science GPA: 3.14; Mean MCAT: (9.0 VR, 9.0. PS, 10.0 BS, N/A); Deadline: Dec. 15th

Loyola University Chicago Stritch School of Medicine
2160 South First Avenue
Maywood, IL 60153

http://www.meddean.luc.edu

E-mail	N/A
Phone	(708) 216-3229
Fax	N/A

- Private. Year Organized: 1870. Percent URM: 5; Percent Women: 45; Percent Out-of-State: 50; Mean Entering Age: 23; Estimated Annual Cost: $27,700 (all students).

- Number of Applicants: 8,464; Number Matriculated: 130; Mean GPA: 3.57; Mean Science GPA: 3.50; Mean MCAT: (9.7 VR, 9.7 PS, 10 BS, O); Deadline: Nov. 15th

Northwestern University Medical School
303 East Chicago Avenue

Chicago, IL 60611-3008

http://www.nums.nwu.edu

E-mail   med-admissions@nwu.edu
Phone   (312) 503-8206
Fax   N/A

• Private. Year Organized: 1859. Percent URM: 8; Percent Women: 46; Percent Out-of-State: N/A; Mean Entering Age: 23; Estimated Annual Cost: $29,247 (all students).

• Number of Applicants: 8,715; Number Matriculated: 174; Mean GPA: 3.70; Mean Science GPA: 3.59; Mean MCAT: (10.1 VR, 10.6 PS, 10.9 BS, P); Deadline: Oct. 15th

Rush Medical College of Rush University
600 South Paulina Street
Chicago, IL 60612

http://www.rush.edu

E-mail   N/A
Phone   (312) 942-6913
Fax   (312) 942-2333

• Private. Year Organized: 1837. Percent URM: 10; Percent Women: 44; Percent Out-of-State: 15-20; Mean Entering Age: N/A; Estimated Annual Cost: $25,824 (all students).

• Number of Applicants: 5,609; Number Matriculated: 120; Mean GPA: 3.23; Mean Science GPA: 3.14; Mean MCAT: (9.0 VR, 9.0 PS, 10.0 BS, N/A); Deadline: Nov. 15th

Southern Illinois University School of Medicine ♦
801 North Rutledge
P.O. Box 19620
Springfield, IL 62794-9620

http://www.siumed.edu

E-mail   egraham@siumed.edu
Phone   (217) 782-2860
Fax   (217) 785-5538

• Public. Year Organized: 1969. Percent URM: 8; Percent Women: 43; Percent Out-of-State: 5; Mean Entering Age: 22; Estimated Annual Cost: Residents, $9,116; s, $27,348.

• Number of Applicants: 1,792; Number Matriculated: 72; Mean GPA: 3.55; Mean Science GPA: 3.53; Mean MCAT: (9.4 VR, 8.8 PS, 9.6 BS, O); Deadline: Nov. 15th

University of Chicago Division of the Biological Sciences The Pritzker School of Medicine ♦ ‡
5841 South Maryland Avenue, MC1000
Chicago, IL 60637-1470

http://www.bsd.uchicago.edu

E-mail   N/A
Phone   (773) 702-1937
Fax   (773) 702-2598

- Private. Year Organized: N/A. Percent URM: 10; Percent Women: 45; Percent Out-of-State: 65; Mean Entering Age: 25; Estimated Annual Cost: $23,880 (all students).

- Number of Applicants: 7,965; Number Matriculated: 104; Mean GPA: 3.62; Mean Science GPA: 3.65; Mean MCAT: (10.2 VR, 10.7 PS, 10.5 BS, N/A); Deadline: Nov. 15th

University of Illinois College of Medicine ♦ ‡
Post Office Box 6998
(M/C 784)
Chicago, IL 60680

http://www.uic.edu/depts/mcam

E-mail   med-admit@mailbox.comd.vic.edu
Phone   (312) 996-5635
Fax   (312) 996-6693

- Public. Year Organized: 1881. Percent URM: 20; Percent Women: 40; Percent Out-of-State: 10; Mean Entering Age: N/A; Estimated Annual Cost: Residents, $13,936; s, $36,782.

- Number of Applicants: 4,468; Number Matriculated: 286; Mean GPA: 3.44; Mean Science GPA: 3.34; Mean MCAT: (9.6 VR, 9.7 PS, 9.8 BS, N/A); Deadline: Dec. 31st

INDIANA
Indiana University School of Medicine
Indiana University Medical Center
1120 South Drive
Indianapolis, IN 46202-5114

http://www.medicine.iu.edu

E-mail   N/A
Phone   (317) 274-3772
Fax   N/A

- Public. Year Organized: 1903. Percent URM: 6; Percent Women: 38; Percent Out-of-State: 5; Mean Entering Age: N/A; Estimated Annual Cost: Residents, $12,370; s, $29,150.

- Number of Applicants: 2,135; Number Matriculated: 280; Mean GPA: 3.67; Mean Science GPA: N/A; Mean MCAT: (9.5 VR, 9.7 PS, 10.0 BS, N/A); Deadline: Dec. 15th

IOWA
University of Iowa College of Medicine
200 Medicine Administration Building
Iowa City, IA 52242-1101

http://www.medadmin.uiowa.edu/osac/admiss.html

E-mail   medical-admissions@uiowa.edu
Phone   (319) 335-8052
Fax   (319) 335-8049

• Public. Year Organized: 1850. Percent URM: 8; Percent Women: 44; Percent Out-of-State: 18; Mean Entering Age: N/A; Estimated Annual Cost: Residents, $9,416; s, $25,220.

• Number of Applicants: 2,556; Number Matriculated: 175; Mean GPA: 3.60; Mean Science GPA: 3.60; Mean MCAT: (9.5 VR, 9.5 PS, 9.5 BS, N/A); Deadline: Nov. 1st

KANSAS
University of Kansas School of Medicine
3901 Rainbow Boulevard
Kansas City, KS 66160-7300

http://www.kumc.edu/som/som.html

E-mail   N/A
Phone   (913) 588-5245
Fax   (913) 588-5259

• Public. Year Organized: 1899. Percent URM: 14; Percent Women: 40; Percent Out-of-State: 5; Mean Entering Age: 26; Estimated Annual Cost: Residents, $9,660; s, $22,818.

- Number of Applicants: 1,408; Number Matriculated: 175; Mean GPA: 3.60; Mean Science GPA: 3.50; Mean MCAT: (9.0 VR, 9.0 PS, 9.0 BS, O); Deadline: Oct. 15th

KENTUCKY
University of Kentucky College of Medicine
MN-150
Chandler Medical Center
Lexington, KY 40536-0298

http://www.comed.uky.edu/medicine

E-mail	N/A
Phone	(606) 323-6161
Fax	(606) 323-2076

- Public. Year Organized: 1956. Percent URM: 6; Percent Women: 38; Percent Out-of-State: 10; Mean Entering Age: 23; Estimated Annual Cost: Residents, $9,150; s, $22,910.

- Number of Applicants: 1,471; Number Matriculated: 97; Mean GPA: 3.59; Mean Science GPA: 3.55; Mean MCAT: (9.25 VR, 9.43 PS, 9.73 BS, O); Deadline: Nov. 1st

University of Louisville School of Medicine
Abell Administration Center
323 East Chestnut Street
Louisville, KY 40202-3866

http://www.louisville.edu/medschool

E-mail   medadm@louisville.edu
Phone   (502) 852-5193
Fax   (502) 852-0302

• Public. Year Organized: 1833. Percent URM: 9; Percent Women: 49; Percent Out-of-State: 10; Mean Entering Age: N/A; Estimated Annual Cost: Residents, $11,166; s, $28,094.

• Number of Applicants: 1,452; Number Matriculated: 141; Mean GPA: 3.59; Mean Science GPA: 3.53; Mean MCAT: (8.9 VR, 9.0 PS, 9.1 BS, N/A); Deadline: Nov. 1st

LOUISIANA
Louisiana State University School of Medicine in New Orleans
1542 Tulane Avenue
New Orleans, LA 70112-2822

http://www.lsuhsc.edu

E-mail   ms-admissions@lsumc.edu
Phone   (504) 568-6262
Fax   (504) 568-7701

• Public. Year Organized: 1931. Percent URM: 15; Percent Women: 41; Percent Out-of-State: 0; Mean Entering Age: 23; Estimated Annual Cost: Residents, $6,549; s, $20,069.

- Number of Applicants: 1,315; Number Matriculated: 167; Mean GPA: N/A; Mean Science GPA: 3.40; Mean MCAT: (8.9 VR, 8.4 PS, 8.6 BS, N/A); Deadline: Nov. 15th

Louisiana State University School of Medicine in Shreveport
Post Office Box 33932
Shreveport, LA 71130-3932

http://www.sh.lsumc.edu

E-mail   shvadm@lsumc.edu
Phone   (318) 675-5190
Fax   (318) 675-5244

- Public. Year Organized: 1969. Percent URM: 5; Percent Women: 33; Percent Out-of-State: 0; Mean Entering Age: N/A; Estimated Annual Cost: Residents, $6,551; s, $20,069.

- Number of Applicants: 1,046; Number Matriculated: 100; Mean GPA: 3.50; Mean Science GPA: 3.40; Mean MCAT: (9.0 VR, 8.4 PS, 8.9 BS, N/A); Deadline: Nov. 15th

Tulane University School of Medicine
1430 Tulane Avenue
New Orleans, LA 70112

http://www.mcl.tulane.edu

E-mail   medsch@tmcpop.tmc.tulane.edu

Phone   (504) 588-5187
Fax   (504) 599-6735

• Private. Year Organized: 1834. Percent URM: 12; Percent Women: 45; Percent Out-of-State: 78; Mean Entering Age: 24; Estimated Annual Cost: $28,275 (all students).

• Number of Applicants: 8,439; Number Matriculated: 150; Mean GPA: 3.50; Mean Science GPA: 3.53; Mean MCAT: (9.9 VR, 10.0 PS, 10.1 BS, P); Deadline: Dec. 15th

MASSACHUSETTS
Boston University School of Medicine
715 Albany Street
Boston, MA 02118

http://www.bumc.bu.edu

E-mail   N/A
Phone   (617) 638-4630
Fax   N/A

• Private. Year Organized: 1848. Percent URM: 10; Percent Women: 38; Percent Out-of-State: N/A; Mean Entering Age: 24; Estimated Annual Cost: $34,250 (all students).

• Number of Applicants: 10,065; Number Matriculated: 143; Mean GPA: 3.58; Mean Science GPA: 3.55; Mean MCAT: (9.41 VR, 9.94 PS, 10.36 BS, N/A); Deadline: Nov. 15th

Harvard Medical School
25 Shattuck Street
Boston, MA 02115

http://www.hms.harvard.edu

E-mail   hmsadm@warren.med.harvard.edu
Phone   (617) 432-1550
Fax   (617) 432-3307

• Private. Year Organized: 1782. Percent URM: 18; Percent Women: 45; Percent Out-of-State: N/A; Mean Entering Age: N/A; Estimated Annual Cost: $26,000 (all students).

• Number of Applicants: 3,463; Number Matriculated: 165; Mean GPA: 3.8; Mean Science GPA: N/A; Mean MCAT: (10.8 VR, 12.0 PS, 11.9 BS, N/A); Deadline: Oct. 15th

Tufts University School of Medicine ‡
136 Harrison Avenue
Boston, MA 02111

http://www.tufts.edu/med

E-mail   N/A
Phone   (617) 636-6571
Fax   N/A

• Private. Year Organized: 1893. Percent URM: 11; Percent Women: 41; Percent Out-of-State: 72; Mean Entering Age: N/A; Estimated Annual Cost: $32,865 (all students).

• Number of Applicants: 9,338; Number Matriculated: 168; Mean GPA: N/A; Mean Science GPA: N/A; Mean MCAT: (9.1 VR, 9.6 PS, 9.8 BS, N/A); Deadline: Nov. 1st

University of Massachusetts Medical School
55 Lake Avenue North
Worcester, MA 01655-0112

http://www.ummed.edu

E-mail   anne.parlante@banyan.ummed.edu
Phone   (508) 856-2323
Fax   N/A

• Public. Year Organized: N/A. Percent URM: 7; Percent Women: 51; Percent Out-of-State: 0; Mean Entering Age: 25; Estimated Annual Cost: Residents, $8,352; s, N/A.

• Number of Applicants: 814; Number Matriculated: 100; Mean GPA: N/A; Mean Science GPA: 3.50; Mean MCAT: (10.0 VR, 10.0 PS, 10.0 BS, N/A); Deadline: Nov. 1st

MARYLAND
Johns Hopkins University School of Medicine
720 Rutland Avenue

Baltimore, MD 21205

http://www.med.jhu.edu/admissions

E-mail   N/A
Phone   (410) 955-3182
Fax   N/A

• Private. Year Organized: N/A. Percent URM: 10; Percent Women: 47; Percent Out-of-State: N/A; Mean Entering Age: N/A; Estimated Annual Cost: $24,500 (all students).

• Number of Applicants: 3,290; Number Matriculated: 118; Mean GPA: N/A; Mean Science GPA: N/A; Mean MCAT: (N/A VR, N/A PS, N/A BS, N/A); Deadline: Nov. 1st

Uniformed Services University of the Health Sciences F. Edward Hebert School of Medicine
4301 Jones Bridge Road
Bethesda, MD 20814-4799

http://www.usuhs.mil

E-mail   N/A
Phone   (301) 295-3101
Fax   (301) 295-3545

• Private (military). Year Organized: 1972. Percent URM: 3; Percent Women: 23; Percent Out-of-State: N/A; Mean Entering Age: 24; Estimated Annual Cost: No tuition.

- Number of Applicants: 2,916; Number Matriculated: 165; Mean GPA: 3.55; Mean Science GPA: 3.54; Mean MCAT: (9.9 VR, 10.2 PS, 10.5 BS, O); Deadline: Nov. 1st

University of Maryland School of Medicine
655 West Baltimore Street
Baltimore, MD 21201

http://www.som1.umaryland.edu

E-mail   N/A
Phone   (410) 706-7478
Fax   N/A

- Public. Year Organized: 1807. Percent URM: 20; Percent Women: 48; Percent Out-of-State: 14; Mean Entering Age: N/A; Estimated Annual Cost: Residents, $12,543; s, $24,301.

- Number of Applicants: 3,806; Number Matriculated: 141; Mean GPA: 3.66; Mean Science GPA: N/A; Mean MCAT: (9.6 VR, 9.8 PS, 10.1 BS, N/A); Deadline: Nov. 1st

MICHIGAN
Michigan State University College of Human Medicine
A-110 East Fee Hall
East Lansing, MI 48824

http://www.chm.msu.edu

E-mail   mdadmissions@msu.edu
Phone   (517) 353-9620
Fax   (517) 432-0021

• Public. Year Organized: N/A. Percent URM: 27; Percent Women: 52; Percent Out-of-State: 20; Mean Entering Age: 25; Estimated Annual Cost: Residents, $16,400; s, $35,000.

• Number of Applicants: 3,404; Number Matriculated: 106; Mean GPA: N/A; Mean Science GPA: N/A; Mean MCAT: (9.7 VR, 8.6 PS, 9.1 BS, N/A); Deadline: Nov. 15th

University of Michigan Medical School
1301 Catherine Road
Medical Science Building I
Ann Arbor, MI 48109-0624

http://www.med.umich.edu/medschool

E-mail   N/A
Phone   (734) 764-6317
Fax   (734) 763-0453

• Public. Year Organized: 1817. Percent URM: 15; Percent Women: 41; Percent Out-of-State: 45; Mean Entering Age: N/A; Estimated Annual Cost: Residents, $18,200; s, $27,950.

- Number of Applicants: 5,114; Number Matriculated: 144; Mean GPA: 3.60; Mean Science GPA: N/A; Mean MCAT: (10.0 VR, 11.0 PS, 11.0 BS, N/A); Deadline: Nov. 15th

Wayne State University School of Medicine
540 East Canfield Avenue
Detroit, MI 48201

http://www.med.wayne.edu

E-mail	N/A
Phone	(313) 577-1466
Fax	(313) 577-1330

- Public. Year Organized: 1868. Percent URM: 18; Percent Women: 55; Percent Out-of-State: 12; Mean Entering Age: N/A; Estimated Annual Cost: Residents, $10,739; s, $21,812.

- Number of Applicants: 32,998; Number Matriculated: 254; Mean GPA: 3.60; Mean Science GPA: N/A; Mean MCAT: (8.8 VR, 9.1 PS, 8.8 BS, N/A); Deadline: Dec. 15th

MINNESOTA
Mayo Medical School
200 First Street, S.W.
Rochester, MN 55905

http://www.mayo.edu/education/mms/MMS_home _page.html

E-mail	N/A
Phone	(507) 284-3671
Fax	(507) 284-2634

- Private. Year Organized: N/A. Percent URM: 15; Percent Women: 51; Percent Out-of-State: N/A; Mean Entering Age: N/A; Estimated Annual Cost: $22,440 (all students).

- Number of Applicants: 3,800; Number Matriculated: 43; Mean GPA: 3.70; Mean Science GPA: 3.80; Mean MCAT: (11.0 VR, 11.0 PS, 11.0 BS, N/A); Deadline: Nov. 1st

University of Minnesota Medical School—Twin Cities
Mayo Mail Code 293
420 Delaware Street S.E.
Minneapolis, MN 55455

http://www.med.umn.edu

E-mail	galva001@maroon.tc.umn.edu
Phone	(612) 624-1122
Fax	(612) 626-4200

- Public. Year Organized: 1888. Percent URM: 2; Percent Women: 47; Percent Out-of-State: 11; Mean Entering Age: N/A; Estimated Annual Cost: Residents, $17,976; s, $33,396

- Number of Applicants: 1,945; Number Matriculated: 165; Mean GPA: 3.60; Mean Science GPA: 3.60; Mean MCAT: (10.0 VR, 10.0 PS, 9.0 BS, N/A); Deadline: Nov. 15th

University of Minnesota—Duluth School of Medicine
10 University Drive
Duluth, MN 55812

http://www.d.umn.edu/medweb

E-mail   jcarls10@d.umn.edu
Phone   (218) 726-8511
Fax   (218) 726-6235

• Public. Year Organized: 1972. Percent URM: 19; Percent Women: 56; Percent Out-of-State: 4; Mean Entering Age: N/A; Estimated Annual Cost: Residents, $16,540; s, $30,768.

• Number of Applicants: 949; Number Matriculated: 53; Mean GPA: 3.60; Mean Science GPA: 3.50; Mean MCAT: (9.1 VR, 8.9 PS, 9.4 BS, N/A); Deadline: Nov. 15th

MISSOURI
Saint Louis University School of Medicine
1402 South Grand Boulevard
St. Louis, MO 63104

http://www.slu.edu/colleges/med

E-mail   mcpeters@slu.edu
Phone   (314) 577-8205
Fax   (314) 577-8214

- Private. Year Organized: 1818. Percent URM: 5; Percent Women: 46; Percent Out-of-State: 64; Mean Entering Age: N/A; Estimated Annual Cost: $27,140 (all students).

- Number of Applicants: 6,206; Number Matriculated: 151; Mean GPA: 3.70; Mean Science GPA: 3.60; Mean MCAT: (9.4 VR, 9.9 PS, 10.2 BS, N/A); Deadline: Dec. 15th

University of Missouri-Columbia School of Medicine
MA204 Medical Sciences Building
One Hospital Drive
Columbia, MO 65212

http://www.muhealth.org/~medicine

E-mail	NolkeJ@health.missouri.edu
Phone	(573) 882-2923
Fax	(573) 884-4808

- Public. Year Organized: 1872. Percent URM: 4; Percent Women: 47; Percent Out-of-State: 0; Mean Entering Age: 23; Estimated Annual Cost: Residents, $15,189; s, $29,830.

- Number of Applicants: 920; Number Matriculated: 96; Mean GPA: 3.74; Mean Science GPA: 3.68; Mean MCAT: (9.61 VR, 9.81 PS, 10.13 BS, O); Deadline: Nov. 1st

University of Missouri-Kansas City School of Medicine✶

2411 Holmes Street
Kansas City, MO 64108-2792

http://www.med.umkc.edu

E-mail   N/A
Phone   (816) 235-1870
Fax   (816) 235-5277

• Public. Year Organized: 1969. Percent URM: 6; Percent Women: 55; Percent Out-of-State: 14; Mean Entering Age: 18; Estimated Annual Cost: Residents, $20,059; s, $40,642.

• Number of Applicants: 737; Number Matriculated: 133; Mean GPA: N/A; Mean Science GPA: N/A; Mean MCAT: (N/A VR, N/A PS, N/A BS, N/A); Deadline: Nov. 15th

Washington University School of Medicine
660 South Euclid Avenue
P. O. Box 8106
St. Louis, MO 63110

http://medschool.wustl.edu

E-mail   wumscoa@msnotes.wustl.edu
Phone   (314) 362-6857
Fax   (314) 362-4658

• Private. Year Organized: 1891. Percent URM: 9; Percent Women: 50; Percent Out-of-State: N/A; Mean Entering Age: N/A; Estimated Annual Cost: $29,670 (all students).

• Number of Applicants: 5,133; Number Matriculated: 121; Mean GPA: 3.80; Mean Science GPA: 3.80; Mean MCAT: (11.1 VR, 12.3 PS, 12.4 BS, N/A); Deadline: Nov. 15th

MISSISSIPPI

University of Mississippi School of Medicine
2500 North State Street
Jackson, MS 39216

http://www.umsmed.edu

E-mail   N/A
Phone   (601) 984-5010
Fax   (601) 984-5008

• Public. Year Organized: 1903. Percent URM: 9; Percent Women: 31; Percent Out-of-State: 0; Mean Entering Age: 24; Estimated Annual Cost: Residents, $6,638; s, $12,638.

• Number of Applicants: 597; Number Matriculated: 100; Mean GPA: 3.62; Mean Science GPA: 3.59; Mean MCAT: (9.3 VR, 9.2 PS, 9.3 BS, O); Deadline: Nov. 1st

NEBRASKA

Creighton University School of Medicine

2500 California Plaza
Omaha, NE 68178

http://www.creighton.edu

E-mail   medschadm@creighton.edu
Phone   (402) 280-2798
Fax   (402) 280-1241

• Private. Year Organized: 1892. Percent URM: 19; Percent Women:
  43; Percent Out-of-State: 82; Mean Entering Age: N/A; Estimated
  Annual Cost: $28,010 (all students).

• Number of Applicants: 4,669; Number Matriculated: 115; Mean
  GPA: 3.73; Mean Science GPA: 3.60; Mean MCAT: (9.9 VR, 9.9
  PS, 10.0 BS, Q); Deadline: Dec. 15th

University of Nebraska College of Medicine
986545 Nebraska Medical Center
Omaha, NE 68198-6545

http://www.unmc.edu/UNCOM

E-mail   jmeyers@unmc.edu
Phone   (402) 559-2259
Fax   (402) 559-4148

• Public. Year Organized: 1880. Percent URM: 3; Percent Women: 49;
  Percent Out-of-State: 13; Mean Entering Age: N/A; Estimated
  Annual Cost: Residents, $11,922; s, $23,051.

• Number of Applicants: 907; Number Matriculated: 123; Mean GPA: 3.70; Mean Science GPA: 3.70; Mean MCAT: (9.7 VR, 9.6 PS, 10.2 BS, N/A); Deadline: Nov. 1st

NEVADA
University of Nevada School of Medicine
2040 W. Charleston Blvd., #400
Las Vegas, NV 89102

http://www.unr.edu/unr/med.html

E-mail	asa@unr.edu
Phone	(702) 784-6063
Fax	(702) 784-6194

• Public. Year Organized: N/A. Percent URM: 5; Percent Women: 43; Percent Out-of-State: 7; Mean Entering Age: 24; Estimated Annual Cost: Residents, $7,483; s, $21,292.

• Number of Applicants: 925; Number Matriculated: 46; Mean GPA: 3.50; Mean Science GPA: 3.40; Mean MCAT: (9.3 VR, 8.8 PS, 9.3 BS, N/A); Deadline: Nov. 1st

NEW HAMPSHIRE
Dartmouth Medical School ‡
Hanover, NH 03755-3833

http://www.dartmouth.edu/dms

E-mail   N/A
Phone   (603) 650-1505
Fax   (603) 650-1614

- Private. Year Organized: N/A. Percent URM: 12; Percent Women: 46; Percent Out-of-State: N/A; Mean Entering Age: 23; Estimated Annual Cost: $23,260 (all students).

- Number of Applicants: 6,687; Number Matriculated: 72; Mean GPA: 3.40; Mean Science GPA: 3.60; Mean MCAT: (10.0 VR, 10.0 PS, 10.0 BS, N/A); Deadline: Nov. 1st

NEW JERSEY
UMDNJ—New Jersey Medical School
185 South Orange Avenue
Newark, NJ 07103-2714

http://www.umdnj.edu/njmsweb

E-mail   njms_admiss@umdnj.edu
Phone   (973) 972-4631
Fax   (973) 972-7986

- Public. Year Organized: 1977. Percent URM: 12; Percent Women: 37; Percent Out-of-State: 3; Mean Entering Age: N/A; Estimated Annual Cost: Residents, $15,509; s, $24,270.

- Number of Applicants: 2,910; Number Matriculated: 177; Mean GPA: 3.50; Mean Science GPA: N/A; Mean MCAT: (9.4 VR, 9.7 PS, 9.8 BS, N/A); Deadline: Dec. 1st

University of Medicine and Dentistry of New Jersey Robert Wood Johnson Medical School
675 Hoes Lane
Piscataway, NJ 08854-5635

http://www2.umdnj.edu/rwjms.html

E-mail   N/A
Phone   (732) 235-4576
Fax   (732) 235-5078

- Public. Year Organized: N/A. Percent URM: 12; Percent Women: 42; Percent Out-of-State: N/A; Mean Entering Age: N/A; Estimated Annual Cost: Residents, $14,920; s, $23,350.

- Number of Applicants: 2,767; Number Matriculated: 138; Mean GPA: 3.50; Mean Science GPA: N/A; Mean MCAT: (9.0 VR, 9.4 PS, 9.7 BS, N/A); Deadline: Dec. 1st

NEW MEXICO
University of New Mexico School of Medicine
Albuquerque, NM 87131

http://hsc.unm.edu/som

E-mail   N/A
Phone   (505) 272-4766
Fax   (505) 272-8239

• Public. Year Organized: 1961. Percent URM: 24; Percent Women: 59; Percent Out-of-State: 4; Mean Entering Age: N/A; Estimated Annual Cost: Residents, $6,478; s, $18,572.

• Number of Applicants: 1,179; Number Matriculated: 92; Mean GPA: 3.50; Mean Science GPA: N/A; Mean MCAT: (9.3 VR, 9.3 PS, 9.3 BS, N/A); Deadline: Nov. 15th

NEW YORK
Albany Medical College
Mail Code 34, Room MS-129
47 New Scotland Avenue
Albany, NY 12208

http://www.amc.edu

E-mail   N/A
Phone   (518) 262-5521
Fax   (518) 262-5887

• Private. Year Organized: 1839. Percent URM: 6; Percent Women: 51; Percent Out-of-State: N/A; Mean Entering Age: N/A; Estimated Annual Cost: $29,330 (all students).

- Number of Applicants: 7,859; Number Matriculated: 124; Mean GPA: 3.40; Mean Science GPA: 3.30; Mean MCAT: (9.8 VR, 9.8 PS, 10.2 BS, N/A); Deadline: Nov. 15th

Albert Einstein College of Medicine of Yeshiva University
1300 Morris Park Avenue
Bronx, NY 10461

http://www.aecom.yu.edu

E-mail   admissions@aecom.yu.edu
Phone   (718) 430-2106
Fax   (718) 430-8825

- Private. Year Organized: N/A. Percent URM: 6; Percent Women: 48; Percent Out-of-State: N/A; Mean Entering Age: N/A; Estimated Annual Cost: $27,650 (all students).

- Number of Applicants: 7,954; Number Matriculated: 180; Mean GPA: 3.60; Mean Science GPA: 3.60; Mean MCAT: (9.4 VR, 10.1 PS, 10.0 BS, N/A); Deadline: Nov. 1st

Columbia University College of Physicians and Surgeons ✳
630 West 168th Street
New York, NY 10032

http://www.cpmc.columbia.edu

E-mail   PT8@columbia.edu

Phone   (212) 305-3595
Fax   (212) 305-3544

- Private. Year Organized: 1767. Percent URM: 10; Percent Women: 43; Percent Out-of-State: N/A; Mean Entering Age: 24; Estimated Annual Cost: $28,008 (all students).

- Number of Applicants: 3,727; Number Matriculated: 149; Mean GPA: N/A; Mean Science GPA: N/A; Mean MCAT: (10.6 VR, 11.1 PS, 11.1 BS, N/A); Deadline: Oct. 15th

Joan & Sanford I. Weill Medical College Cornell University
1300 York Avenue
New York, NY 10021

http://www.med.cornell.edu

E-mail   cumc-admissions@mail.med.cornell.edu
Phone   (212) 821-0560
Fax   (212) 821-0576

- Private. Year Organized: 1898. Percent URM: 18; Percent Women: 53; Percent Out-of-State: 49; Mean Entering Age: N/A; Estimated Annual Cost: $26,200 (all students).

- Number of Applicants: 7,081; Number Matriculated: 101; Mean GPA: N/A; Mean Science GPA: 3.63; Mean MCAT: (10.2 VR, 10.9 PS, 11.2 BS, N/A); Deadline: Oct. 15th

Mount Sinai School of Medicine of New York University
One Gustave L. Levy Place
New York, NY 10029-6574

http://www.mssm.edu

E-mail   N/A
Phone   (212) 241-6696
Fax   (212) 828-4135

• Private. Year Organized: 1968. Percent URM: 16; Percent Women: 49; Percent Out-of-State: N/A; Mean Entering Age: 23; Estimated Annual Cost: $22,050 (all students).

• Number of Applicants: 5,430; Number Matriculated: 105; Mean GPA: 3.60; Mean Science GPA: 3.50; Mean MCAT: (9.5 VR, 9.5 PS, 9.5 BS, N/A); Deadline: Nov. 1st

New York Medical College
Administration Building
Valhalla, NY 10595

http://www.nymc.edu

E-mail   N/A
Phone   (914) 594-4507
Fax   (914) 594-4976

• Private. Year Organized: 1860. Percent URM: 8; Percent Women: 47; Percent Out-of-State: N/A; Mean Entering Age: 23; Estimated Annual Cost: $28,150 (all students).

• Number of Applicants: 10,047; Number Matriculated: 188; Mean GPA: 3.50; Mean Science GPA: 3.40; Mean MCAT: (9.7 VR, 10.1 PS, 10.4 BS, N/A); Deadline: Dec. 1st

New York University School of Medicine ✳
550 First Avenue
New York, NY 10016

http://www.med.nyu.edu

E-mail   N/A
Phone   (212) 263-5290
Fax   N/A

• Private. Year Organized: 1841. Percent URM: 7; Percent Women: 44; Percent Out-of-State: N/A; Mean Entering Age: N/A; Estimated Annual Cost: $22,605 (all students).

• Number of Applicants: 4,045; Number Matriculated: 146; Mean GPA: 3.70; Mean Science GPA: N/A; Mean MCAT: (10.5 VR, 11.8 PS, 11.7 BS, N/A); Deadline: Nov. 20th

State University of New York Health Science Center at Brooklyn College of Medicine ‡
450 Clarkson Avenue, Box 97
Brooklyn, NY 11203-2098

http://www.hscbklyn.edu

E-mail   admissions@netmail.hscbkyln.edu
Phone   (718) 270-2446
Fax   (718) 270-7592

• Public. Year Organized: 1860. Percent URM: 11; Percent Women: 49; Percent Out-of-State: 2; Mean Entering Age: 24; Estimated Annual Cost: Residents, $10,840; s, $21,940.

• Number of Applicants: 3,505; Number Matriculated: 180; Mean GPA: 3.60; Mean Science GPA: 3.50; Mean MCAT: (9.0 VR, 10.0 PS, 10.5 BS, N/A); Deadline: Dec. 15th

State University of New York Health Science Center at Syracuse College of Medicine
750 East Adams Street
Syracuse, NY 13210

http://www.hscsyr.edu

E-mail   N/A
Phone   (315) 464-4570
Fax   (315) 464-8867

• Public. Year Organized: 1872. Percent URM: 5; Percent Women: 46; Percent Out-of-State: 7; Mean Entering Age: N/A; Estimated Annual Cost: Residents, $10,840; s, $21,940.

- Number of Applicants: 2,918; Number Matriculated: 153; Mean GPA: N/A; Mean Science GPA: N/A; Mean MCAT: (9.0 VR, 9.0 PS, 9.0 BS, N/A); Deadline: Nov. 1st

State University of New York Health Sciences Center at Stony Brook School of Medicine
Level 4—Room 169
Stony Brook, NY 11794-8430

http://www.hsc.sunysb.edu/som

E-mail   admissions@dean.som.sunsyb.edu
Phone   (516) 444-2113
Fax   (516) 444-6032

- Public. Year Organized: 1971. Percent URM: 9; Percent Women: 45; Percent Out-of-State: 0; Mean Entering Age: 24; Estimated Annual Cost: Residents, $10,840; s, $21,940.

- Number of Applicants: 3,116; Number Matriculated: 100; Mean GPA: 3.60; Mean Science GPA: 3.60; Mean MCAT: (10.0 VR, 11.0 PS, 11.0 BS, N/A); Deadline: Nov. 15th

State University of New York at Buffalo School of Medicine & Biomedical Sciences
3435 Main Street
Buffalo, NY 14214

http://wings.buffalo.edu

E-mail   jrusso@ascu.buffalo.edu
Phone   (716) 829-3467
Fax   (716) 829-3849

• Public. Year Organized: 1846. Percent URM: 11; Percent Women: 51; Percent Out-of-State: 3; Mean Entering Age: N/A; Estimated Annual Cost: Residents, $10,840; s, $21,940.

• Number of Applicants: 2,500; Number Matriculated: 135; Mean GPA: 3.50; Mean Science GPA: 3.50; Mean MCAT: (9.6 VR, 9.7 PS, 9.7 BS, N/A); Deadline: Oct. 15th

University of Rochester School of Medicine and Dentistry
601 Elmwood Avenue
Box 706
Rochester, NY 14642

http://www.urmc.rochester.edu

E-mail   mdadmish@urmc.rochester.edu
Phone   (716) 275-4539
Fax   (716) 273-1016

• Private. Year Organized: 1920. Percent URM: 13; Percent Women: 50; Percent Out-of-State: N/A; Mean Entering Age: 23; Estimated Annual Cost: $25,950 (all students).

- Number of Applicants: 7,005; Number Matriculated: 100; Mean GPA: 3.60; Mean Science GPA: 3.60; Mean MCAT: (10.0 VR, 10.7 PS, 10.6 BS, N/A); Deadline: Oct. 15th

NORTH CAROLINA
Duke University School of Medicine ♦
Post Office Box 3701
Durham, NC 27710

http://www2.mc.duke.edu/depts/som

E-mail   N/A
Phone   (919) 684-2985
Fax   (919) 684-8893

- Private. Year Organized: 1930. Percent URM: N/A; Percent Women: 49; Percent Out-of-State: 84; Mean Entering Age: N/A; Estimated Annual Cost: $26,700 (all students).

- Number of Applicants: 6,049; Number Matriculated: 98; Mean GPA: N/A; Mean Science GPA: N/A; Mean MCAT: (N/A VR, N/A PS, N/A BS, N/A); Deadline: Oct. 15th

The Brody School of Medicine at East Carolina University
Greenville, NC 27858-4354

http://www.med.ecu.edu/deptmenu.htm

E-mail   N/A
Phone   (252) 816-2202
Fax   (252) 816-3192

• Public. Year Organized: 1972. Percent URM: 21; Percent Women: 50; Percent Out-of-State: N/A; Mean Entering Age: 25; Estimated Annual Cost: Residents, $2,132; s, $21,814.

• Number of Applicants: 1,737; Number Matriculated: 67; Mean GPA: 3.50; Mean Science GPA: 3.40; Mean MCAT: (8.4 VR, 8.2 PS, 8.8 BS, N/A); Deadline: Nov. 15th

University of North Carolina at Chapel Hill School of Medicine
Chapel Hill, NC 27599

http://www.med.unc.edu

E-mail   admissions@med.unc.edu
Phone   (919) 962-8331
Fax   N/A

• Public. Year Organized: 1879. Percent URM: 17; Percent Women: 49; Percent Out-of-State: 50; Mean Entering Age: N/A; Estimated Annual Cost: Residents, $2,502; s, $26,500.

• Number of Applicants: 5,859; Number Matriculated: N/A; Mean GPA: N/A; Mean Science GPA: N/A; Mean MCAT: (9.8 VR, 9.1 PS, 9.3 BS, N/A); Deadline: Nov. 15th

Wake Forest University School of Medicine ‡
Medical Center Boulevard
Winston-Salem, NC 27157

http://www.bgsm.edu

E-mail   medadmit@bgsm.edu
Phone   (336) 716-4264
Fax   (336) 716-5807

• Private. Year Organized: 1902. Percent URM: 11; Percent Women: 41; Percent Out-of-State: 40; Mean Entering Age: 23; Estimated Annual Cost: $27,500 (all students).

• Number of Applicants: 5,859; Number Matriculated: 108; Mean GPA: 3.40; Mean Science GPA: 3.40; Mean MCAT: (10.2 VR, 9.9 PS, 10.0 BS, P); Deadline: Nov. 1st

NORTH DAKOTA
University of North Dakota School of Medicine and Health Sciences ✳
501 North Columbia Road
Box 9037
Grand Forks, ND 58202-9037

http://www.med.und.nodak.edu

E-mail   judy.heit@mail.med.und.nodak.edu
Phone   (701) 777-4221
Fax   (701) 777-4942

- Public. Year Organized: 1905. Percent URM: 17; Percent Women: 45; Percent Out-of-State: N/A; Mean Entering Age: 25; Estimated Annual Cost: Residents, $10,050; s, $26,834.

- Number of Applicants: 306; Number Matriculated: 56; Mean GPA: 3.62; Mean Science GPA: N/A; Mean MCAT: (9.0 VR, 9.1 PS, 9.4 BS, O); Deadline: Nov. 1st

OHIO
Case Western Reserve University School of Medicine ⧧
10900 Euclid Avenue
Cleveland, OH 44106-4915

http://mediswww.cwru.edu

E-mail	N/A
Phone	(216) 368-3450
Fax	(216) 368-4621

- Private. Year Organized: N/A. Percent URM: 14; Percent Women: 43; Percent Out-of-State: 40; Mean Entering Age: N/A; Estimated Annual Cost: $28,600 (all students).

- Number of Applicants: 7,308; Number Matriculated: 145; Mean GPA: 3.60; Mean Science GPA: N/A; Mean MCAT: (10.6 VR, 10.6 PS, 10.6 BS, N/A); Deadline: Oct. 15th

Medical College of Ohio
Post Office Box 10008

Toledo, OH 43699-0008

http://www.mco.edu

E-mail   N/A
Phone   (419) 383-4229
Fax   (419) 383-4005

• Public. Year Organized: 1972. Percent URM: 10; Percent Women:
  30; Percent Out-of-State: 20; Mean Entering Age: 23; Estimated
  Annual Cost: Residents, $10,512; s, $22,966.

• Number of Applicants: 3,689; Number Matriculated: 140; Mean
  GPA: 3.51; Mean Science GPA: 3.47; Mean MCAT: (9.42 VR, 9.34
  PS, 9.48 BS, N/A); Deadline: Nov. 1st

Northeastern Ohio Universities College of Medicine
4209 State Route 44
Post Office Box 95
Rootstown, OH 44272-0095

http://www.neoucom.edu

E-mail   admission@neoucom.edu
Phone   (330) 325-6270
Fax   (330) 325-8372

• Public. Year Organized: N/A. Percent URM: 4; Percent Women: 44;
  Percent Out-of-State: 5; Mean Entering Age: 22; Estimated Annual
  Cost: Residents, $11,244; s, $22,488.

- Number of Applicants: 1,104; Number Matriculated: 25; Mean GPA: 3.60; Mean Science GPA: 3.46; Mean MCAT: (9.2 VR, 8.9 PS, 9.3 BS, N/A); Deadline: Nov. 1st

Ohio State University College of Medicine and Public Health
254 Meiling Hall
370 West Ninth Avenue
Columbus, OH 43210-1238

http://www.med.ohio-state.edu

E-mail   admiss-med@osu.edu
Phone   (614) 292-7137
Fax   (614) 292-1544

- Public. Year Organized: 1914. Percent URM: 8; Percent Women: 38; Percent Out-of-State: 20; Mean Entering Age: 22; Estimated Annual Cost: Residents, $11,644; s, $31,667.

- Number of Applicants: 3,576; Number Matriculated: 210; Mean GPA: 3.59; Mean Science GPA: 3.57; Mean MCAT: (9.86 VR, 10.53 PS, 10.7 BS, P); Deadline: Nov. 1st

University of Cincinnati College of Medicine
Post Office Box 670555
Cincinnati, OH 45267-0555

http://www.med.uc.edu

E-mail   N/A
Phone   (513) 558-7314
Fax   (513) 558-1165

• Public. Year Organized: N/A. Percent URM: 11; Percent Women: 37; Percent Out-of-State: 17; Mean Entering Age: N/A; Estimated Annual Cost: Residents, $11,982; s, $21,441.

• Number of Applicants: 4,091; Number Matriculated: 161; Mean GPA: 3.59; Mean Science GPA: 3.47; Mean MCAT: (9.4 VR, 10.1 PS, 10.3 BS, N/A); Deadline: Nov. 15th

Wright State University School of Medicine
Post Office Box 927
Dayton, OH 45401-0927

http://www.med.wright.edu

E-mail   som_saa@desire.wright.edu
Phone   (937) 775-2934
Fax   (937) 775-3322

• Public. Year Organized: 1973. Percent URM: 30; Percent Women: 55; Percent Out-of-State: 10; Mean Entering Age: 23; Estimated Annual Cost: Residents, $10,842; s, $15,345.

• Number of Applicants: 3,123; Number Matriculated: 90; Mean GPA: 3.50; Mean Science GPA: 3.42; Mean MCAT: (8.5 VR, 8.3 PS, 8.9 BS, N/A); Deadline: Nov. 15th

OKLAHOMA
University of Oklahoma College of Medicine
Post Office Box 26901
Oklahoma City, OK 73190

http://www.medicine.ouhsc.edu

E-mail   Dotty-Shaw@ouhsc.edu
Phone   (405) 271-2331
Fax   (405) 271-3032

• Public. Year Organized: N/A. Percent URM: 26; Percent Women: 44; Percent Out-of-State: 15; Mean Entering Age: N/A; Estimated Annual Cost: Residents, $8,684; s, $21,460.

• Number of Applicants: 1,199; Number Matriculated: 151; Mean GPA: 3.59; Mean Science GPA: N/A; Mean MCAT: (9.6 VR, 8.8 PS, 9.0 BS, N/A); Deadline: Oct. 15th

OREGON
Oregon Health Sciences University School of Medicine
3181 S.W. Sam Jackson Park Road
Portland, OR 97201-3098

http://www.ohsu.edu/

E-mail   N/A
Phone   (503) 494-2998

Fax   (503) 494-3400

• Public. Year Organized: 1887. Percent URM: 6; Percent Women: 45; Percent Out-of-State: N/A; Mean Entering Age: 24; Estimated Annual Cost: Residents, $14,400; s, $30,351.

• Number of Applicants: 2,123; Number Matriculated: 96; Mean GPA: 3.60; Mean Science GPA: 3.60; Mean MCAT: (9.0 VR, 10.0 PS, 10.0 BS, N/A); Deadline: Oct. 15th

PENNSYLVANIA
Jefferson Medical College of Thomas Jefferson University ‡
1025 Walnut Street
Philadelphia, PA 19107-5083

http://www.tju.edu

E-mail   JMC.admissions@mail.tju.edu
Phone   (215) 955-6983
Fax   (215) 923-6939

• Private. Year Organized: 1824. Percent URM: 6; Percent Women: 46; Percent Out-of-State: 60; Mean Entering Age: 24.5; Estimated Annual Cost: $30,077 (all students).

• Number of Applicants: 8,000; Number Matriculated: 223; Mean GPA: 3.45; Mean Science GPA: 3.50; Mean MCAT: (9.8 VR, 9.8 PS, 9.8 BS, N/A); Deadline: Nov. 15th

MCP Hahnemann University School of Medicine ‡
2900 Queen Lane
Philadelphia, PA 19129

http://www.mcphu.edu

E-mail   admis@auhs.edu
Phone   (215) 991-8202
Fax   (215) 843-1766

• Private. Year Organized: 1850. Percent URM: 28; Percent Women: 44; Percent Out-of-State: 60; Mean Entering Age: 23; Estimated Annual Cost: $27,500 (all students).

• Number of Applicants: 6,615; Number Matriculated: 235; Mean GPA: 3.60; Mean Science GPA: 3.70; Mean MCAT: (9.16 VR, 9.55 PS, 10.1 BS, N/A); Deadline: Dec. 1st

Pennsylvania State University College of Medicine
500 University Drive
Post Office Box 850
Hershey, PA 17033

http://www.collmed.psu.edu

E-mail   hmcsaff@psu.edu
Phone   (717) 531-8755
Fax   (717) 531-6225

- Public. Year Organized: 1967. Percent URM: 28; Percent Women: 44; Percent Out-of-State: 60; Mean Entering Age: 23; Estimated Annual Cost: Residents, $16,824; s, $24,550.

- Number of Applicants: 6,615; Number Matriculated: 108; Mean GPA: 3.60; Mean Science GPA: 3.65; Mean MCAT: (9.16 VR, 9.55 PS, 10.1 BS, N/A); Deadline: Nov. 15th

Temple University School of Medicine
3400 North Broad Street
Philadelphia, PA 19140

http://www.temple.edu/medschool

E-mail	N/A
Phone	(215) 707-3656
Fax	(215) 707-6932

- Public. Year Organized: 1901. Percent URM: 20; Percent Women: 41; Percent Out-of-State: 40; Mean Entering Age: N/A; Estimated Annual Cost: Residents, $23,130; s, $28,234.

- Number of Applicants: 8,172; Number Matriculated: 182; Mean GPA: 3.40; Mean Science GPA: 3.40; Mean MCAT: (9.6 VR, 10.0 PS, 10.2 BS, N/A); Deadline: Dec. 1st

University of Pennsylvania School of Medicine ♦ ‡
36th and Hamilton Walk
Philadelphia, PA 19104-6055

http://www.med.upenn.edu

E-mail   N/A
Phone   (215) 898-8001
Fax   (215) 573-6645

• Private. Year Organized: 1765. Percent URM: 16; Percent Women: 46; Percent Out-of-State: 76; Mean Entering Age: N/A; Estimated Annual Cost: $28,470 (all students).

• Number of Applicants: 7,465; Number Matriculated: 143; Mean GPA: 3.75; Mean Science GPA: N/A; Mean MCAT: (11.5 VR, 11.5 PS, 11.5 BS, N/A); Deadline: Nov. 1st

University of Pittsburgh School of Medicine
Alan Magee Scaife Hall of the Health Professions
Pittsburgh, PA 15261

http://www.dean-med.pitt.edu

E-mail   admissions@fsl.dean-med.pitt.edu
Phone   (412) 648-9891
Fax   (412) 648-8768

• Public. Year Organized: 1886. Percent URM: 9; Percent Women: 48; Percent Out-of-State: 50; Mean Entering Age: N/A; Estimated Annual Cost: Residents, $20,534; s, $27,724.

• Number of Applicants: 4,716; Number Matriculated: 150; Mean GPA: 3.63; Mean Science GPA: 3.66; Mean MCAT: (9.8 VR, 10.5 PS, 10.8 BS, O); Deadline: Dec. 1st

PUERTO RICO
Ponce School of Medicine
Post Office Box 7004
Ponce, PR 00732

http://www.psm.edu

E-mail   N/A
Phone   (787) 840-2511
Fax   (787) 840-9756

• Public. Year Organized: 1980. Percent URM: N/A; Percent Women: 39; Percent Out-of-State: 26; Mean Entering Age: N/A; Estimated Annual Cost: Residents, $16,973; s, $25,304.

• Number of Applicants: 989; Number Matriculated: 61; Mean GPA: 3.37; Mean Science GPA: N/A; Mean MCAT: (N/A VR, N/A PS, N/A BS, N/A); Deadline: Dec. 15th

Universidad Central del Caribe School of Medicine
Call Box 60-327
Bayamon, PR 00960-6032

http://www.uccaribe.edu

E-mail   N/A
Phone   (787) 740-1611
Fax   (787) 269-7550

• Public. Year Organized: 1976. Percent URM: N/A; Percent Women: 43; Percent Out-of-State: N/A; Mean Entering Age: N/A; Estimated Annual Cost: Residents, $17,000; s, $24,000.

• Number of Applicants: 1,009; Number Matriculated: 60; Mean GPA: 3.30; Mean Science GPA: N/A; Mean MCAT: (N/A VR, N/A PS, N/A BS, N/A); Deadline: Dec. 15th

University of Puerto Rico School of Medicine
Medical Sciences Campus
P.O. Box 365067
San Juan, PR 00936-5067

http://www.rcm.upr.edu

E-mail   raponte@rcmaxp.upr.clu.edu
Phone   (787) 758-2525
Fax   (787) 282-7117

• Public. Year Organized: 1949. Percent URM: N/A; Percent Women: 50; Percent Out-of-State: N/A; Mean Entering Age: 26; Estimated Annual Cost: Residents, $5,000; s, $10,500.

• Number of Applicants: 970; Number Matriculated: 115; Mean GPA: 3.65; Mean Science GPA: N/A; Mean MCAT: (7.0 VR, 7.0 PS, 8.0 BS, N/A); Deadline: Dec. 1st

RHODE ISLAND
Brown University School of Medicine ✳
97 Waterman Street
Providence, RI 02912

http://biomed.brown.edu

E-mail   MedSchool_Admissions@brown.edu
Phone   (401) 863-2149
Fax   (401) 863-2660

- Private. Year Organized: 1764. Percent URM: 14; Percent Women: 53; Percent Out-of-State: N/A; Mean Entering Age: 23; Estimated Annual Cost: $26,893 (all students).

- Number of Applicants: 2,036; Number Matriculated: 65; Mean GPA: 3.52; Mean Science GPA: 3.71; Mean MCAT: (9.89 VR, 9.84 PS, 10.21 BS, P); Deadline: Mar. 1st

SOUTH CAROLINA
Medical University of South Carolina College of Medicine
96 Jonathan Lucas Street
P.O. Box 250617
Charleston, SC 29425

http://www2.musc.edu

E-mail   taylorwl@musc.edu
Phone   (803) 792-3283
Fax   (803) 792-3764

• Public. Year Organized: 1824. Percent URM: 15; Percent Women: 41; Percent Out-of-State: 8; Mean Entering Age: 25; Estimated Annual Cost: Residents, $9,500; s, $23,604.

• Number of Applicants: 2,293; Number Matriculated: 138; Mean GPA: 3.0; Mean Science GPA: N/A; Mean MCAT: (8.0 VR, 8.0 PS, 8.0 BS, N/A); Deadline: Dec. 1st

University of South Carolina School of Medicine
Columbia, SC 29208

http://www.med.sc.edu

E-mail   N/A
Phone   (803) 733-3325
Fax   (803) 733-3328

• Public. Year Organized: 1974. Percent URM: 18; Percent Women: 40; Percent Out-of-State: 2; Mean Entering Age: 26; Estimated Annual Cost: Residents, $8,134; s, $22,540.

• Number of Applicants: 1,330; Number Matriculated: 73; Mean GPA: N/A; Mean Science GPA: N/A; Mean MCAT: (N/A VR, N/A PS, N/A BS, N/A); Deadline: Dec. 1st

SOUTH DAKOTA
University of South Dakota School of Medicine
1400 West 22nd
Sioux Falls, SD 57105-1570

http://www.usd.edu/med/som

E-mail   N/A
Phone   (605) 357-1422
Fax   (605) 357-1538

• Public. Year Organized: 1907. Percent URM: 3; Percent Women: 45; Percent Out-of-State: 3; Mean Entering Age: 23; Estimated Annual Cost: Residents, $9,745; s, $23,343.

• Number of Applicants: 580; Number Matriculated: 50; Mean GPA: 3.54; Mean Science GPA: 3.49; Mean MCAT: (8.7 VR, 8.5 PS, 8.8 BS, N/A); Deadline: Nov. 15th

TENNESSEE
East Tennessee State University James H. Quillen College of Medicine
Post Office Box 70694
Johnson City, TN 37614

http://gcom.etsu.edu

E-mail   sacom@etsu.edu
Phone   (423) 439-6221
Fax   (423) 439-8206

- Public. Year Organized: 1978. Percent URM: 3.3; Percent Women: 50; Percent Out-of-State: N/A; Mean Entering Age: N/A; Estimated Annual Cost: Residents, $9,666; s, $18,614.

- Number of Applicants: 1,574; Number Matriculated: 60; Mean GPA: 3.50; Mean Science GPA: N/A; Mean MCAT: (9.7 VR, 9.3 PS, 9.5 BS, N/A); Deadline: Dec. 1st

Meharry Medical College School of Medicine
1005 D. B. Todd Jr. Boulevard
Nashville, TN 37208

http://www.mmc.edu

E-mail   N/A
Phone   (615) 327-6223
Fax   (615) 327-6228

- Private. Year Organized: 1876. Percent URM: 79; Percent Women: 52; Percent Out-of-State: 78; Mean Entering Age: N/A; Estimated Annual Cost: $20,785 (all students).

- Number of Applicants: 4,640; Number Matriculated: 80; Mean GPA: N/A; Mean Science GPA: N/A; Mean MCAT: (7.7 VR, 7.2 PS, 7.8 BS, N/A); Deadline: Dec. 15th

University of Tennessee, Memphis, College of Medicine
800 Madison Avenue
Memphis, TN 38163

http://www.utmem.edu/medicine

E-mail   N/A
Phone   (901) 448-5559
Fax   (901) 448-1740

• Public. Year Organized: 1851. Percent URM: 15; Percent Women: 39; Percent Out-of-State: 10; Mean Entering Age: 24; Estimated Annual Cost: Residents, $9,718; s, $19,248.

• Number of Applicants: 1,700; Number Matriculated: 165; Mean GPA: 3.60; Mean Science GPA: 3.50; Mean MCAT: (9.2 VR, 9.0 PS, 9.4 BS, O); Deadline: Nov. 15th

Vanderbilt University School of Medicine ‡
21st Avenue South at Garland Avenue
Nashville, TN 37232

http://www.mc.vanderbilt.edu/medschool

E-mail   medsch.admis@mcmail.vanderbilt.edu
Phone   (615) 322-2145
Fax   (615) 343-8397

• Private. Year Organized: N/A. Percent URM: 39; Percent Women: 33; Percent Out-of-State: 49; Mean Entering Age: 22; Estimated Annual Cost: $24,000 (all students).

- Number of Applicants: 4,777; Number Matriculated: 104; Mean GPA: 3.72; Mean Science GPA: 3.74; Mean MCAT: (10.3 VR, 11.5 PS, 11.6 BS, Q); Deadline: Oct. 15th

TEXAS
Baylor College of Medicine
One Baylor Plaza
Houston, TX 77030

http://www.bcm.tmc.edu

E-mail   melodym@bcm.tmc.edu
Phone   (713) 798-4842
Fax   N/A

- Public. Year Organized: N/A. Percent URM: 18; Percent Women: 46; Percent Out-of-State: 20; Mean Entering Age: 23; Estimated Annual Cost: Residents, $6,550; s, $19,650.

- Number of Applicants: 2,734; Number Matriculated: 167; Mean GPA: 3.80; Mean Science GPA: N/A; Mean MCAT: (10.5 VR, 11.0 PS, 11.5 BS, N/A); Deadline: Nov. 1st

Texas Tech University Health Sciences Center School of Medicine ‡ †
3601 4th Street
Lubbock, TX 79430

http://www.ttuhsc.edu

E-mail   N/A
Phone   (806) 743-2297
Fax   (806) 743-2725

- Public. Year Organized: 1969. Percent URM: 24; Percent Women: 38; Percent Out-of-State: 0; Mean Entering Age: 23; Estimated Annual Cost: Residents, $7,214; s, $20,314.

- Number of Applicants: 1,449; Number Matriculated: 120; Mean GPA: 3.56; Mean Science GPA: 3.50; Mean MCAT: (9.58 VR, 9.63 PS, 9.83 BS, N/A); Deadline: Nov. 1st

The Texas A & M University System Health Science Center College of Medicine +
147 Joe H. Reynolds Medical Building
College Station, TX 77843-1114

http://hsc.tamu.edu

E-mail   med-stu-aff@tamu.edu
Phone   (409) 845-7743
Fax   (409) 845-5533

- Public. Year Organized: 1971. Percent URM: 39; Percent Women: 59; Percent Out-of-State: 9; Mean Entering Age: N/A; Estimated Annual Cost: Residents, $6,650; s, $19,650.

- Number of Applicants: 1,419; Number Matriculated: 64; Mean GPA: 3.70; Mean Science GPA: N/A; Mean MCAT: (9.3 VR, 9.6 PS, 10.3 BS, N/A); Deadline: Nov. 1st

University of Texas Medical School at San Antonio †
7703 Floyd Curl Drive
San Antonio, TX 78284-7790

http://www.uthscsa.edu

E-mail   jonesd@uthscsa.edu
Phone   (210) 567-2665
Fax   (210) 567-2685

• Public. Year Organized: 1959. Percent URM: 16; Percent Women:
  52; Percent Out-of-State: 6; Mean Entering Age: 24; Estimated
  Annual Cost: Residents, $6,550; s, $19,650.

• Number of Applicants: 2,795; Number Matriculated: 200; Mean
  GPA: 3.46; Mean Science GPA: N/A; Mean MCAT: (9.0 VR, 9.0
  PS, 9.0 BS, N/A); Deadline: Oct. 15th

University of Texas Southwestern Medical Center at Dallas Southwestern
Medical School †
5323 Harry Hines Boulevard
Dallas, TX 75235

http://www.swmed.edu

E-mail   N/A
Phone   (214) 648-5617
Fax   (214) 648-3289

- Public. Year Organized: N/A. Percent URM: 36; Percent Women: 33; Percent Out-of-State: 10; Mean Entering Age: 24; Estimated Annual Cost: Residents, $6,550; s, $19,650.

- Number of Applicants: 2,815; Number Matriculated: 200; Mean GPA: 3.75; Mean Science GPA: N/A; Mean MCAT: (10.3 VR, 11.3 PS, 11.4 BS, O); Deadline: Oct 15th

University of Texas—Houston Medical School ✝
6431 Fannin Street
Houston, TX 77030

http://www.med.uth.tmc.edu

E-mail   N/A
Phone   (713) 500-5116
Fax   (713) 500-0604

- Public. Year Organized: 1969. Percent URM: 22; Percent Women: 44; Percent Out-of-State: 3; Mean Entering Age: 23; Estimated Annual Cost: Residents, $7,150; s, $20,250.

- Number of Applicants: 2,868; Number Matriculated: 200; Mean GPA: 3.60; Mean Science GPA: N/A; Mean MCAT: (9.2 VR, 9.2 PS, 9.7 BS, O); Deadline: Oct. 15th

University of Texas Medical Branch at Galveston ✝
301 University Boulevard

Galveston, TX 77555

http://www.utmb.edu

E-mail   pwylie@utmb.edu
Phone   (409) 772-3517
Fax   (409) 772-5753

- Public. Year Organized: 1881. Percent URM: 15; Percent Women: 41; Percent Out-of-State: 2; Mean Entering Age: 26; Estimated Annual Cost: Residents, $6,550; s, $19,650.

- Number of Applicants: 2,772; Number Matriculated: 200; Mean GPA: 3.57; Mean Science GPA: N/A; Mean MCAT: (N/A VR, N/A PS, N/A BS, N/A); Deadline: Oct. 15th

UTAH
University of Utah School of Medicine
50 North Medical Drive
Salt Lake City, UT 84132

http://www.med.utah.edu/som

E-mail   deans.admissions@hsc.utah.edu
Phone   (801) 581-7498
Fax   (801) 585-3300

- Public. Year Organized: 1904. Percent URM: 12; Percent Women: 32; Percent Out-of-State: 44; Mean Entering Age: 24; Estimated Annual Cost: Residents, $6,921; s, $15,271.

- Number of Applicants: 1,325; Number Matriculated: 100; Mean GPA: 3.71; Mean Science GPA: 3.66; Mean MCAT: (9.9 VR, 10.2 PS, 10.6 BS, N/A); Deadline: Oct. 15th

VIRGINIA

Eastern Virginia Medical School of the Medical College of Hampton Roads
Post Office Box 1980
Norfolk, VA 23501

http://www.evms.edu

E-mail   kfn@worf.evms.edu
Phone   (757) 446-5812
Fax   (757) 446-5896

- Public. Year Organized: 1973. Percent URM: 7; Percent Women: 44; Percent Out-of-State: 30; Mean Entering Age: 26; Estimated Annual Cost: Residents, $14,500; s, $26,000.

- Number of Applicants: 4,681; Number Matriculated: 102; Mean GPA: 3.41; Mean Science GPA: N/A; Mean MCAT: (10.0 VR, 10.0 PS, 10.0 BS, N/A); Deadline: Nov. 15th

University of Virginia School of Medicine
Health System
Box 395, McKim Hall
Charlottesville, VA 22908

http://www.med.virginia.edu/

E-mail   bab7g@virginia.edu
Phone   (804) 924-5571
Fax   (804) 982-2586

• Public. Year Organized: 1825. Percent URM: 11; Percent Women: 44; Percent Out-of-State: 33; Mean Entering Age: N/A; Estimated Annual Cost: Residents, $13,154; s, $25,135.

• Number of Applicants: 4,430; Number Matriculated: 139; Mean GPA: 3.67; Mean Science GPA: N/A; Mean MCAT: (10.22 VR, 10.86 PS, 11.11 BS, Q); Deadline: Nov. 1st

Virginia Commonwealth University School of Medicine
P.O. Box 980565
Richmond, VA 23298-0565

http://www.medschool.vcu.edu

E-mail   mack@som1.som.vcu.edu
Phone   (804) 828-9629
Fax   (804) 828-1246

• Public. Year Organized: 1838. Percent URM: 10; Percent Women: 43; Percent Out-of-State: 28; Mean Entering Age: 23; Estimated Annual Cost: Residents, $10,134; s, $25,981.

• Number of Applicants: 4,586; Number Matriculated: 170; Mean GPA: 3.44; Mean Science GPA: N/A; Mean MCAT: (9.5 VR, 9.8 PS, 9.9 BS, N/A); Deadline: Nov. 15th

VERMONT
University of Vermont College of Medicine
E109 Given Building
Burlington, VT 05405

http://www.med.uvm.edu

E-mail   N/A
Phone   (802) 656-2154
Fax   N/A

• Public. Year Organized: 1822. Percent URM: 2; Percent Women: 54; Percent Out-of-State: 50; Mean Entering Age: 25; Estimated Annual Cost: Residents, $18,150; s, $31,770.

• Number of Applicants: 6,262; Number Matriculated: 94; Mean GPA: 3.30; Mean Science GPA: 3.23; Mean MCAT: (10.0 VR, 9.0 PS, 10.0 BS, N/A); Deadline: Nov. 15th

WASHINGTON
University of Washington School of Medicine
Seattle, WA 98195-6340

http://www.washington.edu/medical/som

E-mail   askuwsom@u.washington.edu
Phone   (206) 543-7212
Fax   N/A

- Public. Year Organized: 1945. Percent URM: 10; Percent Women: 48; Percent Out-of-State: 7; Mean Entering Age: 26; Estimated Annual Cost: Residents, $8,436; s, $21,864.

- Number of Applicants: 3,082; Number Matriculated: 174; Mean GPA: 3.63; Mean Science GPA: N/A; Mean MCAT: (10.1 VR, 10.5 PS, 10.5 BS, P); Deadline: Nov. 1st

WISCONSIN
Medical College of Wisconsin
8701 Watertown Plank Road
Milwaukee, WI 53226

http://www.mcw.edu

E-mail   medschool@mcw.edu
Phone   (414) 456-8246
Fax   N/A

- Public. Year Organized: 1967. Percent URM: 10; Percent Women: 38; Percent Out-of-State: 51; Mean Entering Age: 26; Estimated Annual Cost: Residents, $16,264; s, $26,355.

- Number of Applicants: 5,939; Number Matriculated: 204; Mean GPA: 3.68; Mean Science GPA: 3.58; Mean MCAT: (10.0 VR, 10.0 PS, 10.0 BS, P); Deadline: Nov. 1st

University of Wisconsin Medical School

1300 University Avenue
Madison, WI 53706

http://www.medsch.wisc.edu

E-mail   N/A
Phone   (608) 263-4925
Fax   (608) 262-2327

- Public. Year Organized: 1907. Percent URM: 14; Percent Women: 47; Percent Out-of-State: 20; Mean Entering Age: 27; Estimated Annual Cost: Residents, $15,106; s, $22,420.

- Number of Applicants: 2,299; Number Matriculated: 143; Mean GPA: 3.67; Mean Science GPA: N/A; Mean MCAT: (9.8 VR, 9.9 PS, 10.1 BS, P); Deadline: Oct. 15th

WEST VIRGINIA
Joan C. Edwards School of Medicine at Marshall University
1600 Medical Center Drive
Huntington, WV 25701-3655

http://musom.marshall.edu

E-mail   warren@marshall.edu
Phone   (304) 696-1738
Fax   N/A

- Public. Year Organized: 1972. Percent URM: 18; Percent Women: 34; Percent Out-of-State: 14; Mean Entering Age: 26; Estimated Annual Cost: Residents, $8,684; s, $21,170.

• Number of Applicants: 1,141; Number Matriculated: 48; Mean GPA: 3.50; Mean Science GPA: 3.50; Mean MCAT: (9.0 VR, 8.5 PS, 9.1 BS, N/A); Deadline: Nov. 15th

West Virginia University School of Medicine ♦
Morgantown, WV 26506

http://www.hsc.wvu.edu/som

E-mail   dhall@wvuhsc1.hsc.wvu.edu
Phone   (304) 293-3521
Fax   (304) 293-7968

• Public. Year Organized: 1902. Percent URM: 3; Percent Women: 31; Percent Out-of-State: 5; Mean Entering Age: 23; Estimated Annual Cost: Residents, $8,334; s, $21,834.

• Number of Applicants: 1,146; Number Matriculated: 88; Mean GPA: 3.66; Mean Science GPA: 3.61; Mean MCAT: (9.1 VR, 9.2 PS, 9.7 BS, O); Deadline: Nov. 15th

♦ Medical Schools Offering Combined M.D./J.D. Degree Programs
‡ Medical Schools Offering Combined M.D./M.B.A. Degree Programs

✳ Applications must be made directly to schools
† Apply through the Texas Medical and Dental Schools Application Service (TMDSAS)

APPENDIX B: U.S. MEDICAL SCHOOLS OFFERING M.D./PhD. PROGRAMS

ALABAMA
University of Alabama School of Medicine*
University of South Alabama

ARIZONA
University of Arizona

ARKANSAS
University of Arkansas

CALIFORNIA
University of California, Davis
University of California, Irvine
University of California, Los Angeles*
University of California, San Diego*
University of California, San Francisco*
Loma Linda
University of Southern California
Stanford*

COLORADO
University of Colorado*

CONNECTICUT
University of Connecticut
Yale*

WASHINGTON D.C.
George Washington
Georgetown
Howard

FLORIDA
University of Florida
University of Miami

GEORGIA
Emory*
Medical College of Georgia
Morehouse

HAWAII
University of Hawaii

ILLIINOIS
Chicago Medical School
University of Chicago-Pritzker*
University of Illinois, Chicago

University of Illinois, Urbana-Champaign
Loyola-Stritch
Northwestern*
Rush

INDIANA
Indiana University

IOWA
University of Iowa*

KANSAS
University of Kansas

KENTUCKY
University of Kentucky
University of Louisville

LOUISIANA
Louisiana State University-New Orleans
Louisiana State University-Shreveport
Tulane

MARYLAND
John Hopkins*
University of Maryland
Uniformed Services

MASSACHUSETTS
Boston University
Harvard*
University of Massachusetts
Tufts*

MICHIGAN
Michigan State University
University of Michigan*
Wayne State

MINNESOTA
Mayo
University of Minnesota-Minneapolis*

MISSISSIPPI
University of Mississippi

MISSOURI
University of Missouri-Columbia
University of Missouri-Kansas City
University of St. Louis*
Washington University*

NEBRASKA
Creighton
University of Nebraska Medical Center

NEVADA
University of Nevada

NEW HAMPSHIRE
Dartmouth

NEW JERSEY
UMDNJ-New Jersey Medical
UMDNJ-Robert Wood Johnson

NEW YORK
Albany
Albert Einstein*
Columbia*
Cornell*
Mount Sinai*
New York Medical
New York University*
University of Rochester*
SUNY-Brooklyn
SUNY-Buffalo
SUNY-Stony Brook*
SUNY-Syracuse

NORTH CAROLINA
Duke*
East Carolina
University of North Carolina
Wake Forest

NORTH DAKOTA
University of North Dakota

OHIO
Case Western Reserve
University of Cincinnati
Medical College of Ohio
Northeastern Ohio
Ohio State University
Wright State

OKLAHOMA
University of Oklahoma

OREGON
University of Oregon

PENNSYLVANIA
Thomas Jefferson University
MCP Hahnemann University
Pennsylvania State
University of Pennsylvania*
University of Pittsburgh
Temple

RHODE ISLAND
Brown

SOUTH CAROLINA
Medical University of South Carolina
University of South Carolina

SOUTH DAKOTA
University of South Dakota

TENNESSEE
East Tennessee
Meharry
University of Tennessee-Memphis
Vanderbilt*

TEXAS
Baylor*
Texas A&M
Texas Tech
University of Texas-Southwestern, Dallas*
University of Texas-Galveston
University of Texas-Houston
University of Texas-San Antonio

UTAH
University of Utah

VERMONT
University of Vermont

VIRGINIA
Eastern Virginia
Medical College of Virginia
University of Virginia*

WASHINGTON
University of Washington

WEST VIRGINA
Marshall
West Virginia University

WISCONSIN
Medical College of Wisconsin
University of Wisconsin

* U.S. Medical Schools offering Medical Scientist Training Programs (MSTP) Supported by National Institutes of Health

Appendix C: Accredited Canadian Medical Schools

ALBERTA
University of Alberta Faculty of Medicine and Dentistry
Edmonton, Alberta
Canada T6G 2R7

http://www.ualberta.ca

E-mail	admissions@med.ualberta.ca
Phone Number	(403) 492-9524
Fax Number	(403) 492-9531

• Public. Year Organized 1913. Estimated Annual Cost: Canadian, $5,408; Non-Canadian: NA.

• Number of Applicants: 1,050; Number Matriculated: 105. Deadline: Nov 1.

University of Calgary Faculty of Medicine
3330 Hospital Drive, N.W.
Calgary, Alberta
Canada T2N 4N1

http://www.ucalgary.ca/UofC/faculties/medicine

E-mail	staylor@ucalgary.ca
Phone Number	(403) 220-4262

Fax Number   (403) 270-2681

• Public. Year Organized 1965. Percent URM: NA; Percent Women: 52; Percent Out-of-State: NA; Mean Entering Age: 24; Estimated Annual Cost: Canadian, $6,550; Non-Canadian, $30,000.

• Number of Applicants 1,320; Number Matriculated: 69; Mean GPA: 3.75; Mean Science GPA: NA; Mean MCAT: (9.54 VR, 10.68 PS, 10.62 BS, P); Deadline: Nov 30.

BRITISH COLUMBIA
University of British Columbia Faculty of Medicine
317-2194 Health Sciences Mall
Vancouver, BC
Canada V6T 1Z3

http://www.medicine.ubc.ca

Phone Number   (604) 822-4482
Fax Number   (604) 822-6061

• Public. Year Organized 1950. Percent URM: NA; Percent Women: 56.7; Percent Out-of-State: NA; Mean Entering Age: 23; Estimated Annual Cost: Canadian, $5,353; Non-Canadian, NA.

• Number of Applicants: 737; Number Matriculated: 120; Mean GPA: NA; Mean Science GPA: NA; Mean MCAT: (9.73 VR, 10.41 PS, 10.78 BS, Q); Deadline: Dec 15.

MANITOBA
University of Manitoba Faculty of Medicine
753 McDermot Avenue
Winnipeg, MB
Canada R3E 0W3

http://www.umanitoba.ca

E-mail	registrar_med@umanitoba.ca
Phone Number	(204) 789-3569
Fax Number	(204) 789-3929

• Public. Year Organized 1883. Estimated Annual Cost: Canadian, $10,620; Non-Canadian, NA.

• Number of Applicants: 385; Number Matriculated: 70. Deadline: Nov 17.

NEWFOUNDLAND
Memorial University of Newfoundland Faculty of Medicine
Health Sciences Centre
Prince Philip Drive
St. John's, NF
Canada A1B 3V6

http://www.med.mun.ca/med

E-mail	munmed@morgan.ucs.mun.ca
Phone Number	(709) 737-6762
Fax Number	(709) 737-6396

- Public. Year Organized 1925. Estimated Annual Cost: Canadian, $6,449; Non-Canadian, $30,000.

- Number of Applicants: 750; Number Matriculated: 60; Mean GPA: NA; Mean Science GPA: NA; Mean MCAT: (9 VR, 9 PS, 9 BS, O); Deadline: Nov 13.

NOVA SCOTIA
Dalhousie University Faculty of Medicine
CRC Building, Room C-205
5849 University Avenue
Halifax, NS
Canada B3H 4H7

http://www2.dal.ca

E-mail	brenda.detienne@tupdean2.med.dal.ca
Phone Number	(902) 494-1083
Fax Number	(902) 494-8884

- Private. Year Organized 1868. Estimated Annual Cost: Canadian, $10,010; Non-Canadian, $10,010.

- Number of Applicants: 551; Number Matriculated: 89; Mean GPA: 3.70; Mean Science GPA: NA; Mean MCAT: (10 VR, 10 PS, 10 BS); Deadline: Nov 15.

ONTARIO
McMaster University School of Medicine ♠
Health Sciences Centre
Room 1B7
1200 Main Street West
Hamilton, ON
Canada L8N 3Z5

http://www-fhs.mcmaster.ca/mdprog

E-mail	mdadmit@fhs.csu.mcmaster.ca
Phone Number	(905) 525-9140 ext. 22235
Fax Number	(905) 527-2707

• Public. Year Organized 1965. Estimated Annual Cost: Canadian, $13,022; Non-Canadian, $32,954.

• Number of Applicants: 2,906; Number Matriculated: 100; Mean GPA: 3.5; Mean Science GPA: NA; Mean MCAT: NA; Deadline: Oct 15.

Queen's University Faculty of Health Sciences ♠
Kingston, ON
Canada K7L 3N6

http://meds-ss10.meds.queensu.ca/medicine

Phone Number	(613) 533-2542
Fax Number	(613) 533-6884

- Public. Year Organized 1854. Estimated Annual Cost: Canadian, $9,901; Non-Canadian $17,501.

- Number of Applicants: 1,418; Number Matriculated: 75; Mean GPA: NA; Mean Science GPA: NA; Mean MCAT: (10.77 VR, 11.60 PS, 11.14 BS); Deadline: Nov 1.

University of Ottawa Faculty of Medicine ♠
451 Smyth Road
Ottawa, ON
Canada K1H 8M5

http://www.uottawa.ca/academic/med

E-mail   admissmd@uottawa.ca
Phone Number   (613) 562-5409
Fax Number   (613) 562-5420

- Public. Year Organized 1945. Estimated Annual Cost: Canadian, $8,181; Non-Canadian, NA.

- Number of Applicants: 1,851; Number Matriculated: 83. Deadline: Oct 15.

University of Toronto Faculty of Medicine ♠
1 King's College Circle
Toronto, ON
Canada M5S 1A8

http://www.library.utoronto.ca/ www/medicine

Phone Number	(416) 978-2717
Fax Number	(416) 971-2163

• Public. Year Organized 1887. Estimated Annual Cost: Canadian, $12,026; Non-Canadian, $24,898.

• Number of Applicants: 1,632; Number Matriculated: 177. Deadline: Oct 15.

University of Western Ontario Faculty of Medicine & Dentistry ♠
Health Sciences Addition
Richmond Street North
London, ON
Canada N6A 5C1

http://www.med.uwo.ca

E-mail	admissions@med.uwo.ca
Phone Number	(519) 661-3744
Fax Number	(519) 661-3744

• Public. Year Organized 1878. Estimated Annual Cost: Canadian, $10,737; Non-Canadian, NA.

• Number of Applicants: 1,847; Number Matriculated: 96; Mean GPA: 3.65 minimum; Mean Science GPA: NA; Mean MCAT: (9 VR, 8 PS, 9 BS, Q); Deadline: Oct 15.

QUEBEC
Laval University Faculty of Medicine
Quebec City, PQ
Canada G1K 7P4

http://www.fmed.ulaval.ca

E-mail	admissions@fmed.ulaval.ca
Phone Number	(418) 656-2131, ext. 2492
Fax Number	(418) 656-2733

• Public. Year Organized 1852. Estimated Annual Cost: Canadian, $5,382; Non-Canadian, $13,977.

• Number of Applicants: 1,525; Number Matriculated: 112. Deadline: Mar 1 (for Quebec residents); Feb 1 (for others).

McGill University Faculty of Medicine
3655 Drummond Street
Montreal, PQ
Canada H3G 1Y6

http://www.med.mcgill.ca

Phone Number	(514) 398-3617
Fax Number	(514) 398-4631

• Public. Year Organized 1829. Estimated Annual Cost: Canadian, $8,729; Non-Canadian, 20,953.

• Number of Applicants: 946; Number Matriculated: 111. Deadline: Variable.

Universite de Montreal Faculty of Medicine
2900 boulevard Edouard-Montpetit
P.O. Box 6128, Succ. Centre-Ville
Montreal, PQ
Canada H3C 3J7

http://www.med.umontreal.ca

E-mail	admed@ere.umontreal.ca
Phone Number	(514) 343-6265
Fax Number	(514) 343-6265

• Public. Year Organized 1877. Estimated Annual Cost: Canadian, $4,014; Non-Canadian, $12,414.

• Number of Applicants 1,859; Number Matriculated: 153. Deadline: Mar 1.

Universite de Sherbrooke Faculty of Medicine
3001 12th Avenue North
Sherbrooke, PQ
Canada J1H 5N4

http://www.usherb.ca

E-mail   admmed@courrier.usherb.ca
Phone Number   (819) 564-5208
Fax Number   (819) 564-5208

- Public. Year Organized 1961. Estimated Annual Cost: Canadian, $5,708; Non-Canadian, $15,308.

- Number of Applicants: 1,401; Number Matriculated: 90. Deadline: Mar 1.

SASKATCHEWAN
University of Saskatchewan College of Medicine
B103 Health Sciences Building
107 Wiggins Road
Saskatoon, SK
Canada S7N 5E5

http://www.usask.ca/medicine

Phone Number   (306) 966-8554
Fax Number   (306) 966-6164

- Public. Year Organized 1926. Estimated Annual Cost: Canadian, $5,825; Non-Canadian, NA.

- Number of Applicants: 470; Number Matriculated: 55. Deadline: Jan 15 (In-province); Dec 1 (Out-of-province).

♠ Apply through the Ontario Medical School Application Service (OMSAS). All other Canadian Schools require applications from AMCAS.

Appendix D: Accredited Osteopathic Medical Schools

ARIZONA
Arizona College of Osteopathic Medicine of Midwestern University (AZCOM)
Office of Admissions, AZCOM
Glendale Campus
19555 N. 59th Avenue
Glendale, AZ 85308

http://www.midwestern.edu/Pages /AZCOM.html

E-mail	rfisher@azwebmail.midwestern.edu
Phone	(888) 247-9277 & (602) 572-3215
Fax	(623) 572-3229

- Private. Year Organized: 1996. Percent URM: 4; Percent Women: 39; Percent Out-of-State: 66; Mean Entering Age: 27; Estimated Annual Cost: $25,500 (all students).

- Number of Applicants: 3,000; Number Matriculated: 125; Mean GPA: 3.34; Mean Science GPA: 3.39; Mean MCAT: (8-9 VR, 8-9 PS, 9 BS, NA); Deadline: Feb 1.

CALIFORNIA
Touro University College of Osteopathic Medicine (TUCOM)
Dr. Donald Haight
Director of Admissions

Touro University College of
Osteopathic Medicine
Mare Island, CA 94592

http://www.tucom.edu

E-mail   haight@touro.edu
Phone   (707) 562-5100 or (888) 887-7336 in CA
           (888) 880-7336 outside of CA

• Private. Year Organized: 1997. Percent URM: 3; Percent Women: 43; Percent Out-of-State: 40; Mean Entering Age: 26; Estimated Annual Cost: Resident, $24,700; $24,700.

• Number of Applicants: 2,576; Number Matriculated: 100; Mean GPA: 3.4; Mean Science GPA: 3.5; Mean MCAT: (8-9 VR, 8-9 PS, 8-9 BS, NA); Deadline: Feb 1.

Western University of the Health Sciences College of Osteopathic Medicine of the Pacific (Western U/COMP)
Office of Admissions
Western University of Health Sciences
College of Osteopathic Medicine of the Pacific
309 E. 2nd Street, College Plaza
Pomona, CA 91766-1854

http://www.westernu.edu

E-mail   admissions@westernu.edu
Phone   (909) 469-5335

Fax   (909) 469-5570

• Private. Percent URM: 10; Percent Women: 45; Percent Out-of-State: 42; Mean Entering Age: 27; Estimated Annual Cost: $25,385 (all students).

• Number of Applicants: 2,915; Number Matriculated: 176; Mean GPA: 3.20; Mean Science GPA: 3.20; Mean MCAT: (8-9 VR, 8-9 PS, 8-9 BS, NA). Deadline: Feb 1.

FLORIDA
Nova Southeastern University College of Osteopathic Medicine (NSUCOM)
Admissions Office
Nova Southeastern University
College of Osteopathic Medicine
3200 S. University Drive
Ft. Lauderdale, FL 33328

http://www.medicine.nova.edu

E-mail
Phone   (954) 262-1101 or 1(800) 356-0026 ext. 1101

• Public/Private; Year Organized: 1979. Percent URM; Percent Women:; Percent Out-of-State:; Mean Entering Age:; Estimated Annual Cost: Resident.

• Number of Applicants: ; Number Matriculated: ; Mean GPA:; Mean Science GPA:; Mean MCAT: (VR, PS, BS,); Deadline: Jan 15.

IOWA

Des Moines University—Osteopathic Medical Center (UOMHS)
Admissions Office
3200 Grand Avenue
Des Moines, IA 50312

http://www.uomhs.edu

E-mail   DOADMIT@UOMHS.EDU
Phone   (515) 271-1450 or (800) 240-2767 ext. 1450
Fax   (515) 271-1578

• Private. Percent: URM 19; Percent Women: 40-45; Percent Out-of-
  State: 75; Mean Entering Age: 23.5; Estimated Annual Cost:
  $23,900 (all students).

• Number of Applicants: 2,600; Number Matriculated: 205; Mean
  GPA: 3.45; Mean Science GPA: 3.40; Mean MCAT: (8-9 VR, 8-9
  PS, 8-9 BS, NA); Deadline: Feb 1.

ILLINIOS

Chicago College of Osteopathic Medicine—A College of Midwestern
University (CCOM)
Midwestern University Office of Admissions
555 31st Street
Downers Grove, Illinois 60515

http://www.midwestern.edu/Pages/CCOM.html

E-mail   admiss@midwestern.edu

Phone   (800) 458-6253 or (630) 969-4400

• Private. Percent URM: 21; Percent Women: 32; Percent Out-of-State: 70; Mean Entering Age: 25-29; Estimated Annual Cost: $25,000 (all students).

• Number of Applicants: 4,000; Number Matriculated: 160; Mean GPA: 3.44; Mean Science GPA: 3.39; Mean MCAT: NA. Deadline: Feb 1.

KENTUCKY

Pikeville College School of Osteopathic Medicine (PCSOM)
Stephen M. Payson
Associate Dean for Student Affairs PCSOM
214 Sycamore Street
Pikeville, KY 04150

http://www.pcsom.pc.edu

Phone   (606) 432-9617

• Private. Year Organized: 1997. Percent URM: NA; Percent Women: 25; Percent Out-of-State: 46; Mean Entering Age: 29.5; Estimated Annual Cost: $22,000 (all students).

• Number of Applicants: 1,798; Number Matriculated: 62; Mean GPA: 3.30; Mean Science GPA: 3.30; Mean MCAT: (8-9 VR, 8-9 PS, 8-9 BS); Deadline: Feb 1.

MAINE
University of New England College of Osteopathic Medicine (UNECOM)
Admissions Office
UNECOM
Hills Beach Road
Biddeford, ME 04005

http://www.une.edu

Phone   (800) 477-4863

• Private. Percent URM: 3-4; Percent Women: 50; Percent Out-of-State: 30 (outside of New England); Mean Entering Age: 27.5; Estimated Annual Cost: $25,000 (all students).

• Number of Applicants: 3,000; Number Matriculated: 115; Mean GPA: 3.40; Mean Science GPA: 3.40; Mean MCAT: (9-10 VR, 9-10 PS, 9-10 BS); Deadline: Jan 2.

MICHIGAN
Michigan State University College of Osteopathic Medicine (MSU-COM)
Director of Admissions
C110 East Fee Hall
MSUCOM
East Lansing, MI 48824

http://www.com.msu.edu

Phone   (517) 353-7740

• Public. Year Organized: 1969; Percent URM: NA; Percent Women: 51; Percent Out-of-State: 8; Mean Entering Age: 25; Estimated Annual Cost: Resident, $15,881; $33,797.

• Number of Applicants: 2,500-3,000; Number Matriculated: 129; Mean GPA: NA; Mean Science GPA: NA; Mean MCAT: (8-9 VR, 8-9 PS, 8-9BS); Deadline: Dec 1.

MISSOURI
Kirksville College of Osteopathic Medicine (KCOM)
Office of Admissions
800 West Jefferson
Kirksville, MO 63501

http://www.kcom.edu

E-mail   admissions@kcom.edu
Phone   (660) 626-2237 or (800) 626-5266 x2237
Fax   (660) 626-2969

• Private. Year Organized: 1892. Percent URM: 1.3; Percent Women: 28.1; Percent Out-of-State: 90.5; Mean Entering Age: 25; Estimated Annual Cost: $24,400 (all students).

• Number of Applicants: 3,054; Number Matriculated: 170; Mean GPA: 3.41; Mean Science GPA: 3.32; Mean MCAT: (9VR, 9 PS, 9-10 BS, O); Deadline: Feb 1.

The University of Health Sciences—College of Osteopathic Medicine
(UHS-COM)
Office of Admissions
1750 Independence Avenue
Kansas City, MO 64106-1453

http://www.uhs.edu

E-mail   admissions@stuser.uhs.edu
Phone   1 (800) 234-4847 or (816) 283-2000
Fax   (816) 283-2484

• Private. Year Organized: 1916; Percent: URM 13; Percent Women:
  42; Percent Out-of-State: 83; Mean Entering Age: 26; Estimated
  Annual Cost: $27,750 (all students).

• Number of Applicants: 3,100; Number Matriculated: 220; Mean GPA:
  NA; Mean Science GPA: 3.44; Mean MCAT: NA. Deadline: Feb 1.

NEW JERSEY
University of Medicine and Dentistry of New Jersey School of
Osteopathic Medicine (UMDNJ-COM)
Admissions Office
One Medical Center Drive
Stratford, NJ 08084

http://www.umdnj.edu

E-mail   som@umdnj.edu
Phone   (856) 566-7050

Fax   (856) 566-6895

• Public. Year Organized: 1976. Percent: URM 23; Percent Women: 49; Percent Out-of-State: 8; Mean Entering Age: 24; Estimated Annual Cost: Resident, $16,052; $25,119.

• Number of Applicants: 2,112; Number Matriculated: 79; Mean GPA: 3.51; Mean Science GPA: 3.43; Mean MCAT: (8-9 VR, 8-9 PS, 8-9 BS); Deadline: Feb 1.

NEW YORK
New York College of Osteopathic Medicine of New York Institute of Technology (NYCOM)
Director of Admissions
NYCOM/NYIT
Old Westbury, NY 11568

http://www.sunp.nyit.edu/schools/nycom/nycom.html

E-mail   mschaefer@iris.nyit.edu
Phone   (516) 686-3747
Fax   (516) 686-3831

• Private. Percent URM: 12; Percent Women: 50; Percent Out-of-State: 15-20; Mean Entering Age: 25; Estimated Annual Cost: $24,000 (all students).

• Number of Applicants: 3,000; Number Matriculated: 250; Mean GPA: 3.20; Mean Science GPA: 3.20; Mean MCAT: (8-9 VR, 8-9 PS, 8-9 BS); Deadline: Feb 1.

OHIO
Ohio University College of Osteopathic Medicine (OUCOM)
Office of Admissions
102 Grosvenor Hall
Athens, OH 45701-2979

http://www.oucom.ohiou.edu

E-mail   http://www.oucom.ohiou.edu/ Admissions.htm
Phone   (740) 593-4313

• Public. Year Organized: 1975. Percent URM: 23; Percent Women: 44; Percent Out-of-State: 11; Mean Entering Age: 24; Estimated Annual Cost: Resident, $12,594; $17,845.

• Number of Applicants: 2,047; Number Matriculated: 150; Mean GPA: 3.49; Mean Science GPA: 3.39; Mean MCAT: (8-9 VR, 8-9 PS, 8-9 BS); Deadline: Jan 2.

OKLAHOMA
Oklahoma State University College of Osteopathic Medicine (OSU/COM)
Admissions Office
1111 West 17th Street
Tulsa, OK 74107

http://www.osu.com.okstate.edu

E-mail   labgood@osu-com.okstate.edu

Phone   (918) 561-8421 or (800) 677-1972
Fax   (918) 561-8250

• Public. Year Organized: 1972. Percent URM: 20; Percent Women: 40; Percent Out-of-State: 15; Mean Entering Age: 26; Estimated Annual Cost: Resident, $9,552; $24,244.

• Number of Applicants: 1,330; Number Matriculated: 88; Mean GPA: 3.49; Mean Science GPA: 3.39; Mean MCAT: (9 VR, 8.44PS, 8.83 BS, O); Deadline: Dec 1.

PENNSYLVANIA
Philadelphia College of Osteopathic Medicine (PCOM)
Office of Admissions
4170 City Ave
Philadelphia, PA 19131

http://www.pcom.edu

E-mail   admissions@pcom.edu
Phone   (800) 999-6998
Fax   215-871-6719

• Private. Percent URM: 8; Percent Women: 27; Percent Out-of-State: 35; Mean Entering Age: 24; Estimated Annual Cost: $21,925 (all students).

• Number of Applicants: 2,872; Number Matriculated: 250; Mean GPA: 3.20; Mean Science GPA: 3.20; Mean MCAT: (8-9 VR, 8-9 PS, 8-9 BS); Deadline: Feb 1.

Lake Erie College of Osteopathic Medicine (LECOM)
Office of Admissions
1858 West Grandview Boulevard
Erie, PA 16509

http://www.lecom.edu

Phone   (814) 866-6641

• Private. Year Organized: 1992. Percent URM: NA; Percent Women: 48; Percent Out-of-State: NA; Mean Entering Age: NA; Estimated Annual Cost: $21,115 (all students).

• Number of Applicants: 3,000; Number Matriculated: 144; Mean GPA: 3.00; Mean Science GPA: 3.00; Mean MCAT: NA; Deadline: Feb 1.

TEXAS
University of North Texas Health Science Center (UNTHSC)—
College of Osteopathic Medicine (TCOM) †
Office of Medical Student Admissions
3500 Camp Bowie Boulevard
Fort Worth, TX 76107-2699

http://www.hsc.unt.edu

E-mail   tcomadmissions@hsc.unt.edu
Phone   (800) 535-TCOM or (817) 735-2204
Fax   (817) 735-2225

• Public. Year Organized: 1970. Percent URM: 3; Percent Women: 51; Percent Out-of-State: 10; Mean Entering Age: 25; Estimated Annual Cost: Resident, $6,550; $19,650.

• Number of Applicants: NA; Number Matriculated: 111; Mean GPA: 3.69; Mean Science GPA: 3.58; Mean MCAT: (8-9 VR, 8-9 PS, 8-9 BS); Deadline: Dec 1.

WEST VIRGINIA
West Virginia School of Osteopathic Medicine (WVSOM)
Director of Admissions
400 North Lee Street
Lewisburg, WV 24901

http://www.wvsom.edu

Phone   (800) 356-7836 or (304) 645-6270

• Public. Year Organized: 1974. Percent URM: 3-4; Percent Women: 42; Percent Out-of-State: 30; Mean Entering Age: 26; Estimated Annual Cost: Resident, $13,070; $32,350.

• Number of Applicants: 1,493; Number Matriculated: 75; Mean GPA: 3.40; Mean Science GPA: 3.35; Mean MCAT: (7.9 VR, 6.9 PS, 7.3 BS); Deadline: Feb 1.

† Apply through the Texas Medical and Dental Schools Application Service (TMDSAS)

APPENDIX E

Sample Curriculum Vitae

187 Maplewood Dr. Oakmore, NV 90210	Phone 213-555-5968 Cell 213-555-2847 E-mail name@college.edu

Albert Einstein

CAREER GOALS	[Define your aspirations to become a physician and include any desire for doing research, obtaining an additional degree, or humanitarian work.] *Example:* To gain acceptance into medical school and continue performing research with an emphasis in forensic toxicology.
EDUCATION	*Example:* 1999 – Present University of Chicago Chicago, IL **Humanities Major / Junior** • Credit Hours = 122 • University GPA = 3.51 Math/Science GPA = 3.34 • Expected Date of Graduation: May 2003 • MCAT (April 2002), Total Score (9 VR, 10 PS, O WS, 10 SB)
RESEARCH & WORK EXPERIENCE	*Examples:* Summer 2000 University Clinic Los Angeles, CA **Specimen Transporter** • 40 Hours per Week • Duties: To transfer patient specimens from all parts of the hospital to the laboratory. 2000-2001 Howard University Washington D.C. **Undergraduate Research Assistant** • Mentor: Dr. Jennifer Brown • Department of Molecular Biology • Emphasis: Characterization of cis-Acting Elements Controlling the Transcription of the beta 2 Gene.
EXTRACURRICULAR ACTIVITIES	[Include any organizations you have a major role in, honor societies, and tutoring/mentoring/teaching experiences.] *Examples:* • Premedical AMSA – President 2001 • Golden Key Honor Society • Student Government (Student Affairs Committee)

215

PROFESSIONAL MEMBERSHIPS	[Provide the name of the organization and the years of membership.]
	Example: American Chemical Society (Student Chapter), 2001 American Society of Journalists and Authors, 2002 Society of Professional Photographers, 2003
AWARDS RECEIVED	[Provide the name of the award/scholarship/fellowship and the date it was received.]
	Examples: • University Honors, Fall 2000 & Spring Semester 2001 • Recipient of the Goldstein Scholarship, 2002 • Recipient of the University Research Fellowship, 2003
VOLUNTEER EXPERIENCE	[Provide the name of the organization or institution, department, years of service, and number of hours volunteered.] *Examples:* • St. Luke's Hospital (ER-Radiology), 50 Hours, Spring 2001 • Hope Foundation, 60 Hours, Fall 2001 • The Red Cross, 80, Spring 2002

Publications
[Include any manuscripts, abstracts, and poster presentations. Provide all of the authors in the correct order of publication, title of the work, journal title, volume, and page numbers. Be sure to indicate the status of the paper (e.g. In Progress, Submitted, In Press). Place your name in bold print.]

Examples:
• Gary Coleman, **Albert Einstein**, Keith Richards. *Determination of Pilocarpine Levels of Females under Microgravity.* Journal of Nonsense. 2001, 70:9 1788-1796.
• Mahatma Gandhi, **Albert Einstein**, Darryl Dawkins. *Prevalence and characteristics of great men.* Journal of Great People. (Abstracts). 2002, 11:30.
• Bill Cosby, **Albert Einstein**, Glenn Williams. *Economic evaluation of comedy within third world countries.* 45th Laughter Conference. Poster Presentation. 2003.
• **Albert Einstein**, Fat Albert, Prince Albert, Marv Albert. *The influence of Alberts upon 20th century American culture.* British Journal of Alberts. In Press.

Tips for Writing the Curriculum Vitae
• Have it typed professionally or use appropriate computer software
• Check the spelling of all names of people and institutions
• Print on "resume" quality paper (8 ½" x 11" page size) using gray, ivory, or white
• Make your curriculum vitae early in your academic career and make additions as you continue your educational and extracurricular activities
• Do not be afraid to include achievements because they seem minor to you. They may be impressive to others.
• Include any information that makes you unique

APPENDIX F: TOP RATED SOURCES OF INFORMATION FOR MEDICAL SCHOOL APPLICANTS

General Books on Medicine

Belkin, Lisa. *First, Do No Harm.* Fawcett Books. 1994.

Dirckx, John (Editor); Stedman, Thomas (Editor). *Stedman's Concise Medical Dictionary For The Health Professions.* Williams & Wilkins. 1997.

Gevitz, Norman. *The D.O.'s: Osteopathic Medicine in America.* Johns Hopkins University Press. 1991.

Irving, John. *The Cider House Rules.* Ballantine Books. 1994.

Klass, Perri. *A Not Entirely Benign Procedure: Four Years As a Medical Student.* Plume. 1994.

Konner, Melvin. *Becoming a Doctor: A Journey of Initiation in Medical School.* Penguin USA. 1988.

Lewis S. *Arrowsmith.* New York: Penguin Books. 1924.

London, Oscar. *Kill As Few Patients As Possible.* Ten Speed Pr. 1987.

Marion, Robert. *Learning to Play God: The Coming of Age of a Young Doctor.* Fawcett Books. 1993.

Reynolds, Richard; Stone, John. *On Doctoring: Stories, Poems, Essays.* Simon & Schuster. 1995.

Shem, Samuel. *House of God*. Dell Books. 1981.

Medical School Admissions

American Association of Medical Colleges. *Medical School Admission Requirements, United States and Canada*. Published by the AAMC annually.📖

Goliszek, Andrew. *The Complete Medical School Preparation & Admissions Guide*. Healthnet Press. 2000.

Iserson, Kenneth. *Get Into Medical School: A Guide for the Perplexed*. Galen Press. 1997

Kaufman, Daniel, et al. *Essays That Will Get You Into Medical School*. Barrons Educational. 1998.

The New Physician. American Medical Students Association. Published monthly and free with AMSA membership.

Tysinger, J. *Resumes and Personal Statements for Health Professionals*, 2nd ed. Tucson, AZ:
Galen Press. 1998.

📖 **This book is essential reading for medical school applicants (i.e. you must buy this book).** The annual publication, updated each spring, describes U.S. and Canadian medical schools, including details of entrance requirements for each school, selection factors, curriculum features, current first-year expenses, financial aid information, application and acceptance procedures, and applicant statistics. It includes up-to-date information on medical education, premedical planning, choosing a medical school, the Medical College

Admission Test (MCAT), the American Medical College Application Service (AMCAS), AMCAS-E, financing a medical education, and other aspects of the medical school applicant and admission process. Sections are devoted to information for minority group students and high school students. A chapter on medical schools offering combined college and M.D. degree programs for high school students also is included. Updated each spring.

MCAT Preparation

Amin, Chirag, et al. *Jumpstart MCAT.* Lippincott, Williams & Wilkins. 1997.

Bresnick, Stephen and Bresnick, William. 1997. *Columbia Review MCAT Verbal Reasoning Powerbuilder.* Lippincott, Williams & Wilkins.

Bresnick, Stephen and Bresnick, William. 1997. *Columbia Review MCAT Practice Tests.*
Lippincott, Williams & Wilkins.

MCAT Comprehensive Review, 2000 ed./ by Kaplan. Simon & Schuster. 1999.

MCAT Interpretive Manual: A Guide for Understanding and Using MCAT Scores for Admissions Decisions. Published by the AAMC. 1997.

MCAT Student Manual. Published by the AAMC. 1995.

MCAT Practice Test II; III; IV; V; VI. Published by the AAMC. (1991; 1995; 1998; 2000; 2001)

Yazdani, Shahrad. *AudioLearn: MCAT*. BDS Educational Innovations Inc. 2000.

Internet Sites

American Association of Colleges of Osteopathic Medicine (AACOM): www.aacom.org

American Association of Colleges of Osteopathic Medicine Application Service (AACOMAS): http://aacom.org/students/application.html

America's Best Medical Schools: www.usnews.com/usnews.edu/beyond/grad/gradmed.htm

American Board of Medical Specialties (ABMS): www.abms.org

American Medical Student Association (AMSA) Premed: www.amsa.org/premed

Association of American Medical Colleges (AAMC): www.aamc.org

FinAid: The Financial Aid Information Page: www.finaid.com

Financial Aid from the U.S. Department of Education: www.ed.gov/offices/OSFAP/Students

Free Student Application for Student Aid (FAFSA): www.fafsa.ed.gov

Kaplan Review: www.kaplan.com

Medical School Interview Feedback: www.interviewfeedback.com

Medschool.com: www.medschool.com

MCAT Practice Online: www.e-mcat.com

National Health Service Corps Scholarship Program:
www.bphc.hrsa.gov/nhsc

Official Medical College Admission Test (MCAT) Website:
www.aamc.org/mcat

Ontario Medical School Application Service (OMSAS): www.ouac.on.ca

Princeton Review: www.review.com

Texas Medical and Dental Schools Application Service:
http://dpweb1.dp.utexas.edu/mdac/

The Student Doctor Network: www.studentdoctor.net

ABOUT THE AUTHOR

Aashish R. Parikh is currently a medical student at The University of Texas Health Science Center at San Antonio. He graduated from The University of Texas at Austin in 1999 with a Bachelor of Arts in Biochemistry with Special Honors. Aashish has performed extensive research in the fields of analytical chemistry, cellular/molecular biology, and emergency medicine. Subsequently, he has published numerous journal articles and abstracts concerning forensic toxicology. His goal is to become a physician with an emphasis in international medicine. During medical school, Aashish has been involved with healthcare in the countries of India and Nepal.

0-595-23058-X